7-DAY

APPLE CIDER VINEGAR

DETOX

Recipes

Your Quick-Start Guide to Losing 15LBS in 7-Days and Jumpstarting your Journey to Permanent Weight Loss

By

Kim Cox

The 7-Day Apple Cider Vinegar Cleanse Recipes

Copyright © 2019, By: *Kim Cox*

ISBN: 978-1-950772-21-6

All Rights Reserved. No part of this publication may be reproduced in any form or by any means, including scanning, photocopying, or otherwise without prior written permission of the copyright holder.

Disclaimer:

The information provided in this book is designed to provide helpful information on the subjects discussed. The publisher and author are not responsible for any specific health or allergy needs that may require medical supervision and are not liable for any damages or negative consequences from any treatment, action, application or preparation, to any person reading or following the information in this book.

The 7-Day Apple Cider Vinegar Cleanse Recipes

Table of Contents

INTRODUCTION 7
   CLEANSE AND RESET 7

The 7-Day Apple Cider Vinegar Cleanse 9

Breakfast Recipes 9
   Instant Pot Steel-Cut Oats Recipe 9
   Coconut Flour Waffle Recip 10
   Pineapple Upside-Down Cake Recipe 11
   Pizza Stir Fry Recipe 13
   Coconut Flour Pancakes Recipe 15
   Easy Almond Flour Pancakes 17
   Bacon Broccoli Quiche Recipe 18
   Coconut Flour Apple Cinnamon Muffins 20
   Gluten-Free Zucchini Bread Recipe 21
   Grain-Free Pumpkin Bread and Muffins 22
   Protein-Packed Crepes Recipe (with Cottage Cheese) 23
   Coconut Flour Lemon Blueberry Muffins Recipe 25
   Cheesy Breakfast Casserole Recipe 27
   Coconut Flour Biscuits Recipe 29
   Grain Free Flatbread Recipe with Spinach and Egg 30
   Grain Free Pumpkin Pancakes Recipe 31
   Easy Zucchini Fritters Recipe 32
   Avocado Breakfast Bake Recipe 34
   Breakfast Burger Recipe 35
   "Brain Power" Smoothie Recipe 36
   Grain Free Banana Bread & Muffins 37

DINNER AND LUNCH RECIPES 38
   Blackened Salmon 38
   Pineapple Salsa 39
   Southwestern Quinoa Salad 40
   Cilantro Lime Chicken Burgers 42
   Fattoush Salad 43

The 7-Day Apple Cider Vinegar Cleanse Recipes

- Mezze Platter 45
- Baked Pita Chips 46
- Falafel Bowls (Homemade Cava Bowls) 47
- Healthy Pasta Salad 49
- Avocado Corn Salad 50
- Curry Chicken Salad 51
- Easy Mediterranean Orzo Salad 52
- Deconstructed Guacamole Salad 54
- Kale and Cabbage Salad 55
- Lemon Garlic Chicken + Veggies Sheet Pan Meal 56
- Healthy Easy Kung Pao Chicken 58
- Turkey Eggplant Casserole 60
- Cheesy Broccoli Quinoa Casserole 62
- Naan Pizza with Butternut Squash and Pesto 64
- Butternut Squash Fries 66
- Goat Cheese Stuffed Dates 67
- Mediterranean Salmon Salad 68
- Asian Tofu Tacos 70
- Asian Slaw 71
- Baked Peanut Tofu 73
- Butternut Tofu Sheet Pan Dinner 75
- Baked Sweet Potato Fries 77
- One Pan Roasted Veggie and Chicken Sausage 78
- Pear Salad with Walnuts, Avocado and Grilled Chicken 80
- Healthy Sweet Potato Fries Recipe 82
- Healthy Onion Rings Recipe 83
- Shrimp & Cucumber Appetizers 85
- Easy Zucchini Fritters Recipe 86
- Healthy Chocolate Chip Cookies Recipe 88
- Chia Seed Energy Bars Recipe 90

Snacks 92

- Chocolate Coconut Energy Bars Recipe 92

Kale Chips Recipe 94
Snow Cream Recipe 95
Homemade Fruit Snacks Recipe.. 96
Lactation Cookies Recipe (Gluten Free) 98
Radish Cream Cheese Dip Recipe 100
Smoked Salmon Dip Recipe 101
Strawberry Fruit Leather Recipe (with Beets).. 102

DRINKS AND SMOOTHIES 103

Green Immunity Smoothie.. 103
Two seconds chia pudding smoothie 104
Almond fig and strawberry smoothie 105
Mango peach matcha smoothie 106
Matcha cranberry Christmas smoothie bowl 107
Coconut dessert smoothie 108
Green fruits and basil smoothie 109
Banana 'n berries quinoa smoothie 110
Celery apple berry smoothie... 111
Golden Smoothie to mark a golden milestone 112
Masala chai iced coconut drink... 113
Cold brewed French Earl Grey iced tea... 115
Green bliss greens smoothie with mango and peach 116
Cold brewed French Earl Grey iced tea... 117
The perfect summer smoothie 118
Delicious afternoon pick me up: coconut berry smoothie 119
Lettuce be healthy breakfast smoothie 120
Apple rosemary and cinnamon ice tea 121
Pineapple Beet Juice 122
Blueberry yogurt protein smoothie 123
Mint, ginger and citrus green smoothie 124
Kale and passion fruit smoothie 125
Anti-inflammatory fruit boost infused with rosemary 126
Simple matcha latte {dairy & sugar free}.. 127

Kale loquat green smoothie 128

INTRODUCTION

CLEANSE AND RESET

A body cleanse as you know helps the body rid itself of toxic substances. The body has natural means of doing this through the urine, liver, sweat and feces, completing a body cleanse further helps the liver neutralize toxins and release them from your body. There is a big difference between a cleanse and a detox, although the terms are often used interchangeably. While a detox diet eliminates unhealthy foods from your diet and allows you to eat certain foods with detoxifying properties, a cleanse on the other hand not only eliminates unhealthy foods but concentrates on eating whole, healthy foods to give your palette and eating habits a reset.

However, cleanses are popular these days, and there are dozens to choose from out there. But more than just a passing fad, a body cleanse is a means to rid your body of unnecessary toxins and give it an overall reset. If you always experience issues with digestion, a cleanse can offer some reprieve by eliminating acid and alkaline for faster relief. There are also various other parts of the body that can gain from doing a cleanse, leaving you feeling invigorated as a whole. While there is no such thing as a one-day miracle diet (or any quick fix to reaching your weight loss goal), it can be beneficial to hit the reset button every once in a while, giving you a little push towards feeling better stat and making healthier long-term decisions.

Furthermore, most cleanses claim that unspecified toxins — from nonorganic foods, environmental pollution, and other chemical contaminants — are wreaking havoc on our bodies, taxing our digestive systems, and leading to weight gain and serious ailments. Drinking lots of water is also a major component in many popular cleanses and detoxes.

Fuel yourself with food! It will jumpstart your metabolism after a night of sleep. When you doing a mini-cleanse, I will advise you to skip the bread, cereal or any version of them at breakfast as they will cause your body to retain more water, and instead focus your attention on protein, which will provide satiety. An egg-and-salmon scramble is a perfect combination of protein and metabolism-boosting omega-3s to start the day. Or preferably if you're on the go, opt instead for an easy gut healthy smoothie.

Finally, make sure to eat breakfast, lunch, dinner and at least one snack (absolutely no skipping meals!) and ensure they consist of whole, real foods only. Eating consistently throughout the day will help you build the foundation for ongoing healthy eating. I'm talking loads of veggies, lean protein such as chicken, eggs, grass-fed steak, fish, and healthy fats from nuts, seeds or olives, avocado or coconut.

Remember that doing a cleanse can leave you feeling rejuvenated and renewed. In the onset, you may be adjusting to the removal of certain foods from your diet, and any effects it produces. But once you complete yours cleanse, I assure you that you are bound to feel the positive benefits, both mentally and physically.

The 7-Day Apple Cider Vinegar Cleanse

Breakfast Recipes

Instant Pot Steel-Cut Oats Recipe

Tip:

This is a simple breakfast recipe that will keep you feeling full all morning.

Prep Time 5 mins

Cook Time 28 mins

Course: Breakfast

Servings: 8 cups

Ingredients

- 2 cups of steel-cut oats
- 2 cinnamon sticks (it is optional)
- 6 cups of water
- 1 teaspoon of salt

Directions:

1. First, in the Instant Pot, mix together the oats, water, salt, and cinnamon sticks if using.
2. After which you put on the lid and set the vent to sealing.
3. After that, cook at high pressure for about 3 minutes.
4. Then, let pressure release naturally and serve.

Notes

Feel free to add 2 peeled and chopped apples to the oats before cooking for additional flavor.

Coconut Flour Waffle Recipe

Tip:

This recipe is a protein and fiber rich waffle

Course Breakfast

Prep Time 5 minutes

Cook Time 10 minutes

Servings 6 waffles

Ingredients

- ½ cup of butter or better still coconut oil (melted)
- 1 teaspoon of vanilla extract
- ½ cup of coconut flour
- 8 eggs
- 1 Tablespoon of cinnamon
- ½ teaspoon of salt

Directions:

1. Meanwhile, heat waffle iron; in a medium size bowl beat the eggs with whisk or immersion blender.
2. After which you add the melted butter or coconut oil, vanilla, cinnamon, and salt and mix well.
3. After that, add the coconut flour and mix well. (NOTE: the batter should be thick, but if it is too thin, I suggest you add a little more coconut flour).
4. Then, spoon into preheated and greased waffle iron and cook until light brown and firm to touch.
5. Finally, serve with a pat of butter and some homemade strawberry syrup, pure maple syrup, or preferably almond butter.

Notes

1. Makes about 6 waffles for my size of waffle iron, but may make more or less depending on yours.
2. You can make a big batch of these and freeze for an easy breakfast later. If you want to reheat, all you do is pop them in the toaster or oven.

Pineapple Upside-Down Cake Recipe

Tip:

This recipe is sweet and delicious grain-free pineapple upside down cake with coconut flour and eggs for a protein boost.

Prep Time 20 mins

Cook Time 25 mins

Course: Dessert

Servings: 6 people

Ingredients

- ½ cup of butter or better still coconut oil (softened, but not melted)
- ¼ cup of honey or better still maple syrup (it is optional)
- 1 teaspoon of baking powder
- ¼ cup of fresh cherries (or better still maraschino cherries)
- 2/3 cup of coconut flour
- 8 eggs
- 1 dash salt
- ½ can of cored pineapple slices in juice (or better still ½ of a fresh pineapple)

Directions:

1. Meanwhile, heat oven to 325°F.
2. After which you prepare a 9-inch round baking dish or spring form pan by lining the bottom with parchment paper.

NOTE: if using fresh pineapple, peel, core, and cut into ½ inch slices.

3. After that, arrange the pineapple slices on the bottom of the baking dish you are using.
4. At this point, you place the cherries around and in the center of the pineapple slices.
5. Then, in a medium sized bowl, mix together the butter or coconut oil, coconut flour, eggs, honey or maple syrup, salt, and baking powder to form

a thick dough. If necessary, thin with pineapple juice or preferably coconut milk to get a spreadable consistency.
6. This is when you spread the batter over the pineapple and cherries.
7. Furthermore, bake in the preheated oven for about 25-40 minutes until cooked through and no longer soft in the middle.
8. Finally, loosen the edges of the cake and carefully flip over onto a plate or baking sheet.
9. Serve and enjoy!

Notes

1. if desired, substitute an overripe banana and extra juice to thin in place of the honey or maple syrup.
2. In the other hand, if you are using fresh cherries, you can cook some down with a little water and honey or maple syrup to make a cherry sauce.

Pizza Stir Fry Recipe

Tip:

This is an easy stir fry that kids love! It has all the flavors of pizza with Italian sausage and lots of healthy veggies for a delicious, but guilt-free meal!

Course Main

Prep Time 10 minutes

Cook Time 20 minutes

Servings 9 cups

Ingredients

- 2 medium zucchini (or better still yellow squash)
- 1 large onion
- 10 oz. pepperoni (sliced)
- 2 teaspoons of Italian seasoning
- 1 cup of black olives
- 1 cup of mozzarella or better still Parmesan cheese (shredded, optional)
- 1 lb. Italian sausage
- 1-2 cups of mushrooms
- 2 bell peppers
- 2 cups of fresh spinach
- 2 teaspoons of garlic powder
- ½ cup of banana peppers
- 1 cup of pizza sauce (or pasta sauce)

Directions:

1. First, brown the sausage in a skillet over medium heat until cooked.
2. After that, while the sausage is cooking, peel and dice the zucchini and slice the mushrooms, onion, and bell peppers.
3. At this point, remove the sausage from the pan and set aside.

4. This is when you add the vegetables to the pan and sauté until starting to get tender.
5. Return the sausage to the pan; separate the pepperoni slices and add them to the pan with the sausage and vegetables.
6. Furthermore, slice the black olives and banana peppers and add them to the pan.
7. After which you add the spinach, Italian seasoning, and garlic powder.
8. Then, cook and stir until the spinach is wilted.
9. In addition, warm the sauce in a saucepan on the stove and grate the cheese.
10. Finally, divide the stir fry among bowls, top with sauce and cheese if using.
11. Enjoy!

Notes

I suggest you use whatever combination of vegetables you like best on pizza!

Coconut Flour Pancakes Recipe

Tips:

This recipe is a grain-free coconut flour pancakes that are packed with protein for a healthy and filling breakfast.

Course Breakfast

Prep Time 10 minutes

Cook Time 20 minutes

Servings 12 pancakes

Ingredients

- 1 cup of applesauce
- 1 teaspoon of baking soda
- 2 Tablespoons of honey (it is optional)
- 5 eggs
- ½ cup of coconut flour
- 1 teaspoon cinnamon (it is optional)
- 1 teaspoon vanilla extract (it is optional)

Directions:

1. First, in a medium bowl, mix all ingredients together with a blender, whisk, or immersion blender and let sit 5 minutes to thicken.
2. After which you fold in mix-ins like fresh blueberries if desired.
3. After that, heat a large skillet or pancake griddle.
4. Then, grease skillet or griddle with 1 tablespoon coconut oil or butter.
5. At this point, use a ¼ cup measure to scoop batter onto cooking surface, using the bottom of the measure to spread the pancakes out a little.
6. This is when you cook approximately 3-4 minutes per side until it is browned on the bottom and easy to flip. NOTE: these do take a little longer than "regular" pancakes, so please don't rush them!
7. Furthermore, grease skillet or griddle with additional butter or coconut oil as needed between batches.
8. Finally, top with butter (it makes everything better!) or ghee and enjoy!

Notes

Makes about twelve 4-inch pancakes

Easy Almond Flour Pancakes

Tips:

This recipe is a simple and delicious almond flour pancake with only three necessary ingredients for a fast and healthy breakfast.

Feel free to double or triple for larger groups.

Course Breakfast

Prep Time 5 minutes

Cook Time 5 minutes

Servings 6 -8 pancakes

Ingredients

> 3 eggs
>
> spices such as cinnamon nutmeg, blueberries, vanilla, or other flavors (optional)
>
> 1½ cups of almond flour
>
> 1 cup water or better still milk

Directions:

1. First, mix all ingredients in a medium sized bowl using a hand blender or immersion blender until batter is a pourable consistency.
2. After which you make one test pancake to check for desired thickness and texture.
3. After that, thin with additional water or milk if necessary.
4. Then, cook all pancakes on a preheated griddle or in a large pan for approximately 2-3 minutes until bubbles form.
5. At this point, flip and cook an additional 2-3 minutes until they are done in the center and both sides are golden brown.
6. Enjoy!

Notes

Feel free to play with the add-ins and spices on this one to make your own favorite combo or a delicious seasonal pancake.

Bacon Broccoli Quiche Recipe

Tip:

This crust less bacon broccoli quiche is light and fluffy and packed with flavor.

Course Breakfast, Lunch

Prep Time 30 minutes

Cook Time 50 minutes

Servings 8 people

Ingredients

- 2 cups of broccoli
- 6 eggs
- ¼ teaspoon of black pepper
- 1 cup of milk (or better still almond milk)
- 2 cups of shredded sharp cheddar cheese (optional)
- 6 slices bacon
- 1 small onion
- ½ teaspoon of salt
- ½ teaspoon of garlic powder
- 1 cup of heavy cream (or better still full-fat coconut milk)

Directions:

1. Meanwhile, heat the oven to 375°F.
2. After which you grease a pie plate with coconut oil and set aside.
3. After that, dice the bacon.
4. Then, in a medium-size skillet, cook the bacon until it is cooked, but not yet crispy.
5. Furthermore, while the bacon is cooking chop the broccoli into small, bite-size pieces and finely dice the onion.
6. After which you add the broccoli and onion to the bacon and continue cooking until they are slightly softened.

7. At this point, spread the bacon/broccoli mixture evenly in the bottom of the prepared pie plate.
8. This is when you whisk together the salt, garlic powder, eggs, pepper, milk, and heavy cream in a medium size bowl.
9. In addition, stir in the shredded cheese, if using.
10. After that, pour the egg mixture over the bacon and broccoli.
11. Then, place in the oven and bake for about 45-50 minutes or until a knife inserted near the center comes out clean.
12. Finally, allow the quiche to cool slightly, then slice and enjoy!

Notes

Feel free to eat the quiche warm from the oven or chill it and enjoy it cold.

Coconut Flour Apple Cinnamon Muffins

Course Breakfast

Prep Time 5 minutes

Cook Time 15 minutes

Servings 12

Ingredients

- 1 cup of applesauce
- 2-3 Tablespoons of cinnamon
- 1 teaspoon of vanilla extract
- 2 Tablespoons of honey (or other sweetener of choice)
- 5 eggs
- ½ cup of coconut flour
- 1 teaspoon of baking soda
- ¼ cup of coconut oil

Directions:

1. Meanwhile, heat the oven to 400°F.
2. After which you grease a muffin pan with coconut oil or use silicone muffin cups like these.
3. After that, mix all ingredients in a medium-sized bowl with an immersion blender or whisk until well mixed. **NOTE:** I prefer the immersion blender so the coconut oil mixes evenly even if cold/hard.
4. At this point, let sit 5 minutes. NOTE: This helps the coconut flour absorb moisture and creates a better texture in the finished muffins.
5. Then, use 1/3 cup measure to scoop into muffin tins.
6. Furthermore, bake 12-15 minutes until starting to brown and not soft when lightly touched on the top.
7. Finally, let cool 2 minutes, drizzle with honey (if desired) and serve.

Gluten-Free Zucchini Bread Recipe

Course Breakfast

Prep Time 5 minutes

Cook Time 55 minutes

Servings 12 slices

Ingredients

- ½ cup of butter (or better still ghee melted)
- 2 cups of almond flour
- 7 eggs
- 2 Tablespoons of coconut oil melted
- 1 cup of zucchini grated

Directions:

1. Meanwhile, heat oven to 355°F.
2. After which you line a loaf pan with parchment paper.
3. After that, in a large bowl, beat the eggs with a fork or whisk.
4. Then, mix in the melted butter, coconut oil, and grated zucchini.
5. At this point, add the almond flour and mix until it is a dough-like consistency.
6. Finally, pour into the prepared loaf pan and bake in the preheated oven for about 45-50 minutes or until the edges begin to turn golden brown.

Notes

1. For better result, the best way to grate the zucchini is with a simple box or cheese grater.
2. Remember, if you are cooking at a high altitude, be sure to add another egg to ensure moist, fluffy bread.

Grain-Free Pumpkin Bread and Muffins

Prep Time 5 mins

Cook Time 20 mins

Course: Breakfast

Servings: 12 muffins or 1 loaf

Ingredients

- 1 cup of pumpkin puree
- ½ cup of coconut flour
- 1 teaspoon of vanilla extract
- ¼ cup of honey (or better still a few drops of stevia extract)
- 5 eggs
- ¼ cup of coconut oil (or better still butter softened)
- 1 teaspoon of baking soda
- 1-2 Tablespoons of pumpkin pie spice or better still cinnamon

Directions:

1. Meanwhile, heat oven to 400°F.
2. After which you lightly grease muffin tins or 8x8 baking dish with coconut oil. (**NOTE:** a regular loaf pan doesn't work well)
3. After that, put all ingredients in a medium-sized bowl and mix with an immersion blender or strong whisk until smooth and well incorporated. **NOTE:** if batter is too thick, I suggest you add a little coconut milk or water to thin, but don't let it get runny at all.
4. Then, scoop into greased muffin tins with a ¼ cup measure or pour into a greased 8x8 baking dish.
5. Finally, bake for about 13-18 minutes for muffins or 20-25 minutes for bread until lightly browned and set in middle.

Notes

Optional: To make a crumble topping; finely grind almonds or pecans and mix with butter or coconut oil.

Protein-Packed Crepes Recipe (with Cottage Cheese)

Tip:

These crepes are delicious and healthy, with a hidden boost of protein from lots of cottage cheese and eggs.

Course Breakfast

Prep Time 5 minutes

Cook Time 15 minutes

Servings 16 crepes

Ingredients

- 6 eggs
- 1 teaspoon of salt
- 2 teaspoons of vanilla extract
- 2 Tablespoons of coconut oil for greasing pan
- 2 cups of cottage cheese
- 1 cup of almond flour (or preferably gluten-free flour for a smoother crepe)
- ½ teaspoon of cinnamon
- ¼ + cup of almond milk (or water)

Directions:

1. First, combine all the ingredients except the coconut oil in a blender and blend until smooth.
2. After which you thin with additional almond milk or water if needed to create a smooth and slightly thin batter.
3. Meanwhile, heat a pancake griddle or a skillet on the stove over medium heat, adding a small amount of coconut oil.
4. After that, use a ¼ cup measure to pour batter onto preheated griddle or pan and cook until set in the middle, greasing with additional coconut oil between batches if necessary.

5. Then serve without flipping or for best texture, (carefully) flip and lightly cook the other side.
6. Finally, serve with fresh fruit, honey, peanut butter, or any other desired topping.

Coconut Flour Lemon Blueberry Muffins Recipe

Tips:

This recipe has plenty of protein and healthy fats from coconut flour and pastured eggs.

Course Breakfast

Prep Time 25 minutes

Cook Time 30 minutes

Servings 12 muffins

Ingredients

- ¼ cup of butter (or preferably ghee melted)
- ¼ cup of honey
- 1 Tablespoon of lemon juice
- ½ teaspoon of baking powder
- ½ teaspoon of sea salt
- ½ cup of pecans (it is optional)
- 6 eggs
- ½ cup of coconut milk
- 1 teaspoon of vanilla
- 2/3 cup of coconut flour
- 1 teaspoon of cinnamon
- ½ teaspoon of lemon zest
- 1 cup of fresh or preferably frozen blueberries

Directions:

1. Meanwhile, heat oven to 375°F.
2. After which in a large bowl, blend together melted butter, honey, vanilla, eggs, milk, and lemon juice.

3. After that, in a separate bowl, combine the cinnamon, baking powder, coconut flour, salt, and lemon zest.
4. Then, combine the dry ingredients into the bowl with the eggs and coconut milk until there are no lumps. **NOTE:** Do not over mix.
5. At this point, fold the blueberries into the batter.
6. This is when you allow the batter to sit 5 minutes so that the coconut flour can absorb the liquid.
7. In the meantime, roughly chop the pecans.
8. Furthermore, using a ¼ cup measure, pour the batter into silicone muffin pans or regular pans lined with cupcake liners.
9. After that, top with crushed pecans.
10. Finally, bake for 30 minutes; cool on a wire rack and enjoy!

Notes

Make sure the muffin pans are well greased.

Cheesy Breakfast Casserole Recipe

Course Breakfast

Prep Time 10 minutes

Cook Time 40 minutes

Servings 8 servings

Ingredients

- 6 eggs
- 1 teaspoon of garlic powder
- 8 slices of bacon cooked and crumbled (it is optional)
- 8 oz. cheese of choice grated (it is optional)
- 16 oz. cottage cheese
- ¼ cup of parmesan cheese
- 1 teaspoon of onion powder
- 4 green onions (thinly sliced)

Directions:

1. Meanwhile, heat oven to 350°F.
2. After which you grease a 9X13 baking dish.
3. After that, in a blender or food processor, puree the cottage cheese until smooth.
4. Then, add the parmesan, eggs, garlic powder, and onion powder and pulse until combined.
5. At this point, add the bacon and green onions if using and stir by hand to combine.
6. This is when you pour into greased 9x13 inch dish and bake for about 35-40 minutes or until fork inserted into center comes out clean.
7. Finally, top with cheese and return to oven until just melted. Serve immediately.

Notes

1. This recipe can be made ahead of time and reheated; also try making it in muffin cups for a single serve breakfast, just reduce the cook time to 20 minutes.
2. If you want additional nutrients and fiber, I suggest you mix in chopped spinach or leftover sautéed veggies along with the crumbled bacon and green onions, or serve a salad on the side.

Coconut Flour Biscuits Recipe

Prep Time 5 minutes

Cook Time 15 minutes

Servings 8 biscuits

Ingredients

> 5 Tablespoons of butter or better still coconut oil softened but not melted
>
> 2 Tablespoons of honey (optional)
>
> ½ teaspoon of baking powder
>
> ½ cup of coconut flour
>
> 4 eggs
>
> ½ teaspoon of sea salt

Directions:

1. Meanwhile, heat oven to 400 degrees F.
2. After which you put all ingredients into medium sized bowl and mix well with immersion blender or hand mixer until well incorporated.
3. Furthermore, using your hands, carefully form into eight small balls and gently flatten with a spoon to make it about ½ inch thick.
4. Finally, bake for about 12-15 minutes until just starting to brown.

Notes

When making these the first time, I suggest you add the coconut oil little by little until the consistency seems right.

Grain Free Flatbread Recipe with Spinach and Egg

Course Main

Prep Time 10 minutes

Cook Time 10 minutes

Servings 3 flatbreads

Ingredients

- ¼ cup of arrowroot flour
- 2 Tablespoons of coconut flour
- coconut oil or better still ghee for greasing the pan
- ½ cup of almond flour
- ¼ cup of tapioca flour
- ¾ teaspoon of Himalayan salt
- ½ cup of water

Directions:

1. First, whisk all the flours and salt together.
2. After which you add the water and stir until completely smooth.
3. After that, heat a nonstick skillet over medium heat and lightly grease the pan with a paper towel dipped in coconut oil or ghee.
4. Then, pour a third of the batter into the pan.
5. At this point, let the bread cook and firm up on one side before flipping it over.
6. Furthermore, cook the breads for roughly 2 minutes on each side, then reduce the heat, cover, and cook until firm and golden, taking care not to burn.
7. Finally, repeat for the other two breads.

Notes

You can use the flatbread as a wrap, a pizza crust, or just as you would a piece of toast!

Grain Free Pumpkin Pancakes Recipe

Course Breakfast

Prep Time 5 minutes

Cook Time 10 minutes

Servings 2 servings

Ingredients

- ¼ cup of pumpkin puree GAPS legal canned pumpkin puree or homemade
- Butter honey, maple syrup, or better still fruit butter for serving (optional)
- 2 eggs
- 1/8 teaspoon of cinnamon
- 1 Tablespoon of coconut oil

Directions:

1. First, warm a cast iron pan over medium high heat.
2. After which you whisk together the pumpkin puree, eggs, and cinnamon.
3. After that, add about a Tablespoon of coconut oil to the hot pan and swirl to cover the bottom of the pan.
4. Then, use about two scant Tablespoons of batter for each pancake. (**NOTE:** they flip best when the pancakes are small).
5. At this point, cook until golden on the bottom and slightly opaque in the center and around the edges.
6. Finally, flip, brown on the other side, and serve.
7. This recipe makes about 8 small pancakes, for 1 large serving or 2 medium servings.

Notes

These pancakes do not contain any form of flour at all, so expect it to look a bit thinner than traditional pancakes -- more like a crepe.

Easy Zucchini Fritters Recipe

Tip:

This recipe is easy to make and a great alternative to hash browns and tater tots with an extra nutrient boost!

Course Side

Prep Time 10 minutes

Cook Time 20 minutes

Servings 16 fritters

Ingredients

- 1 teaspoon of salt
- 2 eggs
- ¼ cup of almond flour
- 1 teaspoon of basil leaf
- 2 medium fresh zucchini (or better still 1½ cups frozen shredded zucchini, thawed)
- 1 small onion
- ½ cup of Parmesan cheese (or better still almond flour, or 3 Tablespoons of coconut flour)
- 1 teaspoon of garlic powder
- 1 teaspoon of black pepper

Directions:

1. Meanwhile, heat oven to 400°F.
2. After which you grease a baking sheet or muffin tin.
3. After that, grate the zucchini with a box grater or food processor.
4. Then, add the salt and squeeze very tightly with a towel to get the excess liquid out.
5. At this point, put in a medium sized bowl.
6. This is when you grate the onion and add to the bowl.

7. Furthermore, add the eggs, almond flour, Parmesan cheese, and spices and mix until combined.
8. After that, put Tablespoon size amounts of the mixture onto the baking sheet or fill the muffin tins ½ full.
9. In addition, bake for approximately 18-20 minutes or until tops and sides are starting to brown.
10. Finally, serve alone or with homemade ketchup. NOTE: can also pan fry in coconut oil for a crispier outer coating.
11. Enjoy!

Notes

1. It is time to make your own ketchup!
2. You can store in the refrigerator or freezer.

Avocado Breakfast Bake Recipe

Tips:

This recipe is a creamy avocado baked with an egg for a filling breakfast rich in protein and healthy fats.

Course Breakfast

Prep Time 5 minutes

Cook Time 20 minutes

Servings 2

Ingredients

- 4 eggs
- Feel free to use toppings of choice such as feta and green onions, or salsa and fresh cilantro
- 2 avocados
- salt and pepper

Directions:

1. Meanwhile, heat the oven to 350°F.
2. After which you cut the avocados in half and carefully remove the pit.
3. After that, put avocados open side up in a large baking dish. (**NOTE:** if they are small avocados, scoop out a little of the extra flesh to make more room for the egg).
4. Then, crack one egg into each avocado half and sprinkle with sea salt and pepper.
5. At this point, place in the oven for about 15-20 minutes or until egg is cooked as desired. NOTE: For my oven, 17 minutes gets the perfect egg yolk.
6. Finally, top with desired toppings while still hot and enjoy!

Notes

For the topping; Feel free to come up with your favorite combo!

Breakfast Burger Recipe

Tips:

This recipe is an upgraded version of breakfast sausage with extra nutrients and spices.

Course Breakfast

Prep Time 15 minutes

Cook Time 15 minutes

Servings 24

Ingredients

- 2 pounds of ground pork or preferably ground beef
- 1 teaspoon of black pepper omit on autoimmune program
- 1 teaspoon of dried thyme leaf
- 1 teaspoon of dried fennel (chopped)
- 1 tablespoon of collagen powder
- 1 teaspoon of salt
- 1 teaspoon of dried ground sage
- ½ teaspoon of red pepper flakes omit on autoimmune program
- 1 Tablespoon of maca powder

Directions:

1. First, combine all ingredients in a large bowl and mix well.
2. After which you form into small patties.
3. After that, cook over medium heat in a skillet for about 4 minutes on each side until center is no longer pink. (**NOTE:** for me, I brown the sausage on one side, flip, and add ½ cup of water to the skillet. The steam helps cook the sausage all the way through and prevents sticking).

Notes

You can batch cook these and store in the refrigerator or freezer for quick, easy breakfasts.

"Brain Power" Smoothie Recipe

Tip: this recipe gives you a great energy boost!

Course Drinks

Prep Time 5 minutes

Servings 2

Ingredients

- 1 Tablespoon of MCT oil (or preferably 2 Tablespoons coconut oil)
- ½ teaspoon of vanilla extract
- 1 cup ice
- 1 banana (optional)
- 2 cups of coconut milk
- 2 Tablespoons of gelatin powder
- 2 or more egg yolks
- flavor s of choice such as 1 Tablespoon cocoa powder, ½ cup strawberries, 1 teaspoon cinnamon, etc.

Directions:

First, put all ingredients into blender or Vitamix and blend until smooth.

Grain Free Banana Bread & Muffins

Tip:

This is a tasty grain-free muffin that banana bread lovers will enjoy

Prep Time 5 minutes

Cook Time 13 minutes

Servings 10 muffins

Ingredients

    2 ripe bananas

    ½ cup of coconut flour

    a small amount of milk to thin may not need

    5 eggs

    ¼ cup of coconut oil or better still butter softened

    1 teaspoon of baking soda

    1 teaspoon of vanilla extract

Directions:

1. Meanwhile, heat oven to 400°F.
2. After which you grease muffin tins.
3. After that, put all ingredients in medium sized bowl and whisk using strong whisk or immersion blender.
4. After that, mix until smooth and well incorporated.
5. Furthermore, batter should be thick, but if it is too thick, add a little milk to thin, but don't let it get runny at all.
6. At this point, spoon ¼ cup into each hole of prepared muffin tins.
7. Finally, bake for about 13-18 minutes until lightly browned and set in middle.

Notes

To get the best result, make sure your bananas are good and ripe -- yellow with lots of brown speckles

DINNER AND LUNCH RECIPES

Blackened Salmon

Prep Time: 10 minutes

Cook Time: 10 minutes

Yield: 4

Ingredients

1 Tablespoon of olive oil or butter

pineapple salsa (for serving)

2 cups of white, brown or cauliflower rice, for serving

4 (about 6 oz.) skin-on salmon fillets

3 Tablespoons of blackened seasoning (or better still Cajun seasoning)

Directions:

1. You can make blackened seasoning if needed.
2. First, liberally rub blackened seasoning on the flesh of each salmon fillet.
3. After which you heat oil or butter in a large nonstick or cast iron skillet over medium heat.
4. After that, add the fillets to the skillet, skin-side up, and cook until blackened, about 3 minutes.
5. Then, flip the fillets and continue to cook until they are cooked to your preference, 5 to 7 minutes depending on the thickness of your fillets.
6. Finally, serve over rice and top with pineapple salsa.

Pineapple Salsa

Prep Time: 15 minutes

Total Time: 15 minutes

Yield: 8

Tips:

This recipe is so easy to make!

Feel free to pair it with tortilla chips for a flavorful appetizer or use as a topping for tacos, grilled chicken or fish.

Ingredients

- ¼ cup of finely diced red onion
- 1 jalapeño pepper (seeded and finely diced)
- 2 Tablespoons of fresh cilantro (chopped)
- ½ teaspoon of sea salt
- 1 cup of finely diced pineapple
- ¼ cup of finely diced bell pepper
- 1 clove garlic (minced)
- 1 Tablespoon of lime juice + more to taste

Directions:

1. First, add onion, jalapeño pepper, pineapple, bell pepper, garlic and cilantro in a small bowl.
2. After which you toss with lime juice.
3. After that, taste and add more lime juice if needed.
4. Then, cover and place in the fridge for about 1-2 hours to let the flavors marinate before serving.
5. Finally, serve with tortilla chips as an appetizer or as a topping for fish.

Notes

You can substitute pineapple for fresh mango.

Southwestern Quinoa Salad

Prep Time: 20 minutes

Cook Time: 30 minutes

Yield: 4

Tip:

This recipe is a flavorful and healthy southwestern quinoa salad with roasted sweet potatoes, black beans and avocado.

Ingredients

1 large sweet potato (chopped into bite size chunks)

1 cup of black beans (rinsed and drained)

¼ cup of minced red onion

1 avocado (chopped)

juice of 1 lime

¼ – ½ teaspoon of cayenne

½ sea salt + more to taste

1 cup of uncooked quinoa (rinsed and drained)

1 red or orange bell pepper (cored, seeded, and diced)

1 cup of thawed frozen corn

¼ cup of minced fresh cilantro

¼ cup + ½ Tablespoon of olive oil

1 teaspoon of chili powder

pinch of cumin

ground black pepper (to taste)

Directions:

1. Meanwhile, heat oven to 400°F.
2. After which you toss sweet potato chunks with ½ Tablespoon of olive oil.
3. Season to taste with salt and pepper, and arrange evenly on a baking sheet.

4. After that, bake in the preheated oven until the sweet potatoes are tender, about 25-30 minutes.
5. Then, allow sweet potato chunks to cool.
6. In the meantime, cook the quinoa according to package instructions. Allow quinoa to cool.
7. Furthermore, in a large mixing bowl combine roasted sweet potatoes, corn, black beans, cilantro, quinoa, bell pepper, shallot, and avocado.
8. At this point, add ¼ cup olive oil, chili powder, cumin, lime juice, cayenne, black pepper and sea salt.
9. This is when you gently toss the salad to combine.
10. In addition, taste and adjust the seasoning, if necessary.
11. Then, serve salad right away or chill in the fridge a few hours before serving.
12. Finally, add a sprinkle of queso fresco or feta cheese when serving, if desired.

Cilantro Lime Chicken Burgers

Prep Time: 6 minutes

Cook Time: 14 minutes

Total Time: 20 minutes

Yield: 4

Ingredients

1 Tablespoon of lime juice + 1 teaspoon lime zest

¼ cup of chopped cilantro

½ teaspoon of sea salt

whole wheat or gluten-free hamburger buns or lettuce bun

1 lb. of ground chicken

¼ cup of minced onion

1 teaspoon of garlic powder

Pinch of ground pepper

Toppings of choice: ketchup, jalapeño slices, avocado, red onion, avocado oil mayo

Directions:

1. First, combine all ingredients in a bowl and mix until just combined.
2. After which you shape the mixture into equal sized burgers.
3. After that, spray a little cooking spray on a non-stick skillet or grill pan over medium heat.
4. Then, add burgers to skillet and cook 6-7 minutes per side, or until cooked through and 165°F internally.
5. Finally, serve immediately with toppings and bun of choice.

Fattoush Salad

Prep Time: 20 minutes

Cook Time: 10 minutes

Yield: 6

Tips:

This recipe has vegetables, fresh herbs, crispy pita bread and a bright sumac dressing.

Ingredients

- 2 cups of cherry tomatoes (quartered)
- 1 small head of romaine lettuce (chopped)
- 16 baked pita chips
- 2 cups of mini (or Persian) cucumbers, chopped
- ½ cup of radishes (thinly sliced)
- 1 cup of parsley (chopped)
- ½ cup mint (chopped)

Lemon Dressing

- 3 Tablespoons of lemon juice
- ¼ cup of olive oil
- ¼ teaspoon of black pepper
- 2 cloves of garlic (minced)
- ½ Tablespoon of white balsamic (or preferably white wine vinegar)
- 1 teaspoon of ground sumac
- ½ teaspoon of sea salt

Directions:

1. First, prep and bake pita chips according to the linked recipe; let cool.
2. After which in a bowl whisk together lemon juice, olive oil, garlic, vinegar, sumac, salt, and pepper. Set aside.
3. After that, in a large bowl toss together tomatoes, romaine, cucumbers, radishes, parsley and mint with the lemon dressing.
4. Then, break pita chips into pieces and add half into the bowl with the salad; toss.
5. Finally, plate salad and top each portion with extra broken pita pieces.
6. Make sure you serve immediately.

Notes

1. If you make the full batch of pita chips, you'll have about 8 extra pita chips to snack on later.
2. Remember, feta is totally optional, but it makes a delicious topping for this salad as well!
3. This recipe the veggies and crisp pita are best served fresh.

Mezze Platter

Prep Time: 20 minutes

Yield: 10

Tip:

This Mediterranean snack plate works wonders as an appetizer for potlucks and also dinner parties.

Ingredients

- pita bread or preferably pita chips
- feta
- tabbouleh
- fresh vegetables: bell peppers, chopped carrots, sliced cucumbers,
- cherry or grape tomatoes,
- radishes
- olives
- almonds
- stuffed grape leaves
- Dips of choice: tzatziki, hummus, baba ghanoush (roasted eggplant dip)

Directions:

1. First, arrange all your ingredients on a large platter. **NOTE:** I like starting with bowls for the dips and then covering the rest of the platter with veggies and other snack able items like the feta, olives, stuffed grape leaves, and tabbouleh.
2. Finally, add the pita chips and fresh herbs on top of the dips for a pop of color and decoration.

Baked Pita Chips

Prep Time: 7 minutes

Cook Time: 10 minutes

Yield: 4 servings

Tips:

This recipe is made from just four ingredients.

I bet you that you won't want to go back to store bought pita chips after making these!

Ingredients

- 2 Tablespoons of olive oil
- 1 teaspoon of sea salt
- 3 whole wheat pitas
- 1 teaspoon of garlic powder

Directions:

1. Meanwhile, heat oven to 400°F.
2. After which you cut pita into four wedges, then separate the pita. (NOTE: I found this was easiest to do using kitchen scissors. Remember, that you should end up with a total for 24 triangles).
3. After that, in a small bowl combine the olive oil, garlic powder and sea salt.
4. Then, use a basting brush to brush the oil mixture onto each side of the pita chips.
5. Furthermore, place pita chips on a baking sheet, making sure not to overlap and bake for about 5 minutes, flip and bake for another 5 minutes or until pita is golden and crisp to the touch.
6. Finally, watch carefully because they can burn easily.

Falafel Bowls (Homemade Cava Bowls)

Prep Time: 30 minutes

Cook Time: 24 minutes

Yield: 4 bowls

Tip:

This is recipe is a plant-based Mediterranean meal that you can prep ahead of time for delicious meals all week long.

Ingredients

2 cups of cooked brown rice (or better still cauliflower rice)

1 batch of baked falafel

½ cup of hummus

¼ cup of harissa

¼ cup of pickled onions (it is optional)

pita bread or pita chips (for serving)

4 cups of chopped baby spinach

1 cup of chopped purple cabbage

2 cups of Israeli salad

½ cup of tzatziki

¼ cup of crumbled feta

zesty tahini dressing (to taste)

Directions:

1. First, prep all falafel, hummus, Israeli salad, tzatziki, and tahini dressing by following linked recipes.
2. After which you combine bowls by adding 1 cup chopped baby spinach, ½ cup brown rice, and ¼ cup chopped purple cabbage to each bowl.
3. After that, top each bowl with 3-4 baked falafel patties, 2 Tablespoons tzatziki, ½ cup Israeli salad, 1 Tablespoon harissa, 2 Tablespoons hummus, 1 Tablespoon feta and pickled onions, if using.

4. Then, serve bowls with zesty tahini dressing on the side so each person can add the dressing to taste.
5. Finally, serve with a side of fresh pita bread or baked pita chips.

Notes

1. Harissa is super spicy and might be hard to find, so in that case simply omit it from the recipe.
2. If you prefer more protein, I recommend my apple cider vinegar chicken would be an awesome addition!

Healthy Pasta Salad

Prep Time: 15 minutes

Cook Time: 10 minutes

Yield: 6 cups

Tip:

However, this delicious pasta salad is gluten-free, vegan and perfect for serving a crowd!

Ingredients

- 2 cups of tomatoes (chopped)
- ¾ cup of red onion (chopped)
- 2 Tablespoons of basil (minced)
- ½ teaspoon of coconut sugar
- 1 ½ teaspoons of sea salt
- 8 oz. macaroni or penne pasta (I prefer gluten-free penne)
- 2 cups of cucumbers (peeled and chopped)
- 3 Tablespoons of balsamic vinegar
- 2 Tablespoons of olive oil
- ¼ teaspoon of crushed red pepper

Directions:

1. First, cook pasta according to package instructions.
2. After which you drain and run cold water over cooked pasta to cool.
3. After that, add drained pasta into a large bowl with tomatoes, cucumber, and onion.
4. Then whisk together basil, balsamic vinegar, coconut sugar, olive oil, crushed red pepper and salt.
5. At this point, pour over salad ingredients and mix well.
6. Finally, refrigerate until cold. Serve.

Avocado Corn Salad

Prep Time: 10 minutes

Yield: 8

Tip:

This recipe when topped with lime juice and fresh basil is the perfect healthy summer side dish because there's no cooking involved!

Ingredients

1 cup of red onion (diced)

lime juice (note: 1 lime or about 3 Tablespoons)

Ground pepper (to taste)

6 ears of fresh uncooked sweet corn, husked and cut from cob (about 4 ½ cups)

1 large avocado (diced)

¼ cup of fresh basil (chopped)

1 teaspoon of sea salt

Directions:

1. First, after husking and cutting corn from the cob, pull out as many corn silks as possible.
2. After which you combine all ingredients in a large bowl.
3. After that, serve immediately or allow it to marinate for a few hours. **NOTE:** I like to make it the night before and allow it to marinate over night as it tastes even better the next day.

Notes

1. However, if you prefer to cook the corn, I suggest you fill a large pot with water and bring to a boil.
2. Then, once boiling add corn cobs and boil for 5-6 minutes.
3. After that, remove corn cobs from the boiling water, drain and rinse with cold water.
4. Furthermore, once cool enough to handle, cut corn from the cob.

Curry Chicken Salad

Prep Time: 10 minutes

Yield: 4

Tips:

This recipe with celery, onion and raisins is super flavorful and comes together fast using shredded chicken.

This is an awesome salad to meal prep for lunches throughout the week.

Ingredients

- ¾ cup of celery (chopped)
- ¼ cup of red onion (chopped)
- ½ Tablespoon of curry powder
- ¼ teaspoon of ground pepper
- 2 Tablespoons of cashews (optional)
- 2 cups of shredded chicken
- ¼ –1/3 of cup raisins
- ¼ cup of avocado (or better still olive oil mayonnaise)
- 1 teaspoon of apple cider vinegar
- 1/8– ¼ teaspoon of sea salt

Directions:

1. First, in a large bowl, stir together apple cider vinegar, mayo, curry powder, pepper and salt.
2. After which you add celery, shredded chicken, raisins and red onion to the bowl.
3. After that, stir until well combined.
4. Then, taste and adjust seasonings, if needed.
5. Finally, serve on bread as a sandwich, in lettuce wraps or over a bed of greens.

Easy Mediterranean Orzo Salad

Prep Time: 25 minutes

Cook Time: 10 minutes

Yield: 6

Tips:

This healthy and hearty orzo salad is packed with Mediterranean flavors like sun-dried tomatoes and feta.

In the other hand this is a total crowd-pleaser that you'll want to bring to every summer cookout and potluck.

Ingredients

4 ounces' fresh baby spinach (chopped)

1 cup of diced cucumber

½ cup of cannellini beans (or better still other white bean)

½ cup of crumbled feta cheese

1 cup of uncooked whole wheat orzo pasta

1/3 cup of sun-dried tomatoes (chopped)

10 Kalamata olives (pitted and chopped)

¾ teaspoon of dried oregano

sea salt and black pepper

Balsamic Dressing

1 ½ Tablespoons of maple syrup

1 clove garlic (minced)

3 Tablespoon of olive oil

¼ cup of balsamic vinegar

1 teaspoon of Dijon mustard

½ teaspoon of sea salt

Directions:

1. First, bring a saucepan of water to a boil over high heat.
2. After which you add orzo and cook according to the package directions until just tender, about 8-10 minutes.
3. After that, drain, and rinse under cold water until the pasta cools to room temp.
4. Then, drain well and transfer to a large bowl.
5. Furthermore, while orzo cooks make the dressing by using a blender or whisk to combine all ingredients.
6. At this point, add the cucumber, tomatoes, spinach, olives, beans and oregano to the orzo and toss to combine.
7. This is when you add half of the balsamic dressing and toss again.
8. In addition, taste it and add more dressing if needed.
9. Finally, season with sea salt and black pepper.
10. Make sure you serve at room temperature, sprinkled with feta.

Notes

1. However, you can prep this salad the day before and keep it chilled, covered in the refrigerator.
2. For the best flavor, I suggest you let the chilled salad come to room temperature before serving.

Deconstructed Guacamole Salad

Prep Time: 10 minutes

Yield: 4

Tip:

You can serve this recipe as a healthy side or top with grilled protein for a meal-sized salad.

Ingredients

¼ cup of chopped cilantro

4 roma tomatoes (chopped)

2 avocados (chopped)

¼ cup of sliced red onion

Lime Dressing

Juice of 1 lime

¼ teaspoon of sea salt

2 Tablespoons of olive oil

1 teaspoon of maple syrup

1 clove garlic (minced)

Directions:

1. First, place all ingredients for the dressing in a small jar.
2. After which you shake or stir until everything is combined.
3. After that, taste and add more salt if needed.
4. Then, add ingredients for the salad into a bowl, top with dressing, toss salad and enjoy.

Kale and Cabbage Salad

Prep Time: 20 minutes

Yield: 6

Tip:

This recipe is a lovely kale cabbage salad with broccoli florets, chickpeas and sunflower seeds coated with a creamy nutritional yeast dressing.

Ingredients

- 4 cups of red cabbage (shredded)
- 1 (about 15 oz.) can of chickpeas (drained and rinsed)
- 1 avocado (sliced)
- ¾ cup of nutritional yeast dressing
- 4 cups of kale (approx. 1 bunch), de-stemmed and shredded
- 1 medium crown of broccoli (chopped into bite-size pieces)
- 1/3 cup of roasted unsalted sunflower seeds

Directions:

1. First, make nutritional yeast dressing.
2. After which you chop all your veggies into bite-size pieces and toss into a large bowl to combine.
3. After that, toss in chickpeas and sunflower seeds and top with dressing (Note: I used about ½ the batch, but feel free to add as much or as little as you'd like).
4. Then, use your hands to massage the salad, toss with a large spoon or put a lid on the container and shake until the salad is well coated.

Lemon Garlic Chicken + Veggies Sheet Pan Meal

Prep Time: 10 minutes
Cook Time: 40 minutes
Yield: 4

Ingredients

1 lb. asparagus (trimmed and chopped in half)

1 Tablespoon of olive oil (for potatoes)

1 lb. small potatoes (chopped into bite-size chunks)

1 ½ lb. of boneless skinless chicken breast (chopped into chunks)

Lemon Garlic Sauce

4 cloves garlic (minced)

1 Tablespoon of maple syrup

1 ½ teaspoon of ground pepper

1 teaspoon of dried oregano

juice of 1 lemon

3 Tablespoons of olive oil

1 ½ teaspoon of sea salt

1 teaspoon of dried basil

Directions:

1. Meanwhile, heat oven to 400*F.
2. After which you coat potatoes with 3 Tablespoons of the lemon garlic sauce + an additional Tablespoon of olive oil.

3. After that, roast for 20 minutes.
4. In the meantime, let chicken chunks marinate in remaining sauce.
5. Furthermore, once potatoes have roasted for 20 minutes, toss and add chicken with sauce along with asparagus to the pan.
6. Finally, place pan back in the oven and roast for about 15-25 minutes or until chicken is cooked through.
7. Enjoy warm.

Healthy Easy Kung Pao Chicken

Prep Time: 10 minutes

Cook Time: 15 minutes

Yield: 4

Tips:

This healthy kung pao chicken is packed with nutrients and not lacking any flavor.

It absolutely gluten-free and dairy-free.

Ingredients

- 1 Tablespoon of sesame oil (divided)
- 2 teaspoons of fresh ginger (grated or minced)
- 2 green onions (chopped)
- crushed peanuts, for serving (it is optional)
- 1 lb. boneless skinless chicken breast (chopped into chunks)
- 4 cloves garlic (minced)
- 1 bell pepper (yellow, orange or red), chopped
- 3 cups of broccoli
- 2 cups of cooked brown rice (for serving)

Sauce

- 1–2 Tablespoons of honey
- 1/2–1 teaspoon of arrowroot powder for thickening (optional)
- ¼ cup of coconut aminos (or better still low sodium soy sauce/tamari)
- 2 teaspoons of sambal oelek chili paste or sriracha

Directions:

1. First, make sauce by combining all ingredients in small bowl.

2. After which you heat ½ Tablespoon sesame oil in a large sauté pan or wok.
3. Furthermore, once hot, add chicken, garlic and ginger and cook for about 5-7 minutes until chicken is just cooked through.
4. At this point, transfer chicken to a plate.
5. After that, in the same pan, add remaining oil, green onions, bell pepper, and broccoli and toss.
6. This is when you cook for 5 minutes or until broccoli is tender, then add chicken and sauce to the pan and cook for 2-3 minutes or until sauce thickens a bit.
7. In addition, turn off heat and let rest for 2-3 minutes.
8. After which you serve kung pao chicken and veggies over brown rice.
9. Finally, top with crushed peanuts and sriracha for more spice!

Notes

    a. For me; I prefer using 1 Tablespoon of honey but if you like things on the sweeter side you can add 2 Tablespoons.
    b. Feel free to use cornstarch instead of arrowroot powder if you'd like.
    c. Remember, you can also make the sauce without either.

Turkey Eggplant Casserole

Prep Time: 30 minutes

Cook Time: 40 minutes

Yield: 6

Tips:

This cheesy eggplant casserole layers' eggplant with protein-rich turkey and mozzarella. It bakes up in 30 minutes!

Ingredients

sea salt

1 eggplant (sliced into ¼ inch thick slices)

Turkey Sauce

3 cloves garlic (minced)

1/2 Tablespoon of Italian Seasoning

1 (24 oz.) jar marinara sauce (any flavor)

grated parmesan cheese (to taste)

½ Tablespoon of olive oil

¼ teaspoon of salt and pepper

1 lb. of ground turkey

½ cup of shredded mozzarella cheese

Directions:

1. First, cut eggplant into slices, place on a baking sheet or platter and sprinkle salt on both sides.
2. After which, you let sit for about 20-30 minutes.
3. After that, discard up any water released from the eggplant slices and blot any remaining water with a paper towel.
4. Meanwhile, heat oven to 375°F.
5. Then, heat ½ Tablespoon olive oil in large sauté pan.

6. Furthermore, once hot, add garlic and cook until fragrant, about 2 minutes.
7. After that, add ground turkey into the pan, season with salt, pepper and Italian seasoning.
8. At this point, cook, breaking turkey apart until turkey is cooked through and no longer pink, about 10-15 minutes.
9. Add sauce to the pan and combine; remove from heat.
10. This is when you spray a 9 x 13 baking dish with cooking spray; spread a little sauce into the bottom of the pan and add a layer of eggplant.
11. In addition, top with half the turkey sauce mixture.
12. After which you add another layer of eggplant, top with the remaining turkey sauce mixture.
13. After that, sprinkle on mozzarella cheese.
14. Then, cover eggplant bake with foil and place in preheated oven.
15. Bake for 25 minutes; remove foil and bake for another 5 minutes or until cheese is hot and bubbly.
16. Finally, remove from oven, let rest for 5 minutes and serve.
17. You can serve with grated parmesan.

Cheesy Broccoli Quinoa Casserole

Prep Time: 40 minutes

Cook Time: 15 minutes

Yield: 10

Ingredients

2 cups of water or low sodium broth (for cooking quinoa)

2 Tablespoons of butter

6 cloves garlic (minced)

1 cup milk (I prefer unsweetened almond milk)

1 teaspoon of sea salt

½ teaspoon of garlic powder

1 cup of uncooked quinoa (I prefer Ancient Harvest)

4 cups of fresh broccoli florets

1 ½ cups of chopped yellow onion

2 Tablespoons of oat flour (all-purpose will work too)

8 oz. block of good quality cheddar cheese (divided)

1 teaspoon of ground pepper

Directions:

1. First, lightly coat a casserole dish (I prefer an 8×8 square dish) with non-stick spray or lightly grease.
2. After which you prepare quinoa using water or broth, according to package directions. Note: you should end up with about 3 cups of cooked, fluffy quinoa.
3. After that, place in a large mixing bowl.
4. Furthermore, while quinoa is cooking, steam broccoli for about 5-6 minute or until bright green and crisp tender.
5. In the meantime, shred cheese by using a food processor (affiliate link) with the shredding attachment or with a handheld grater.
6. Meanwhile, heat oven to 350°F.

7. After which you heat butter in a medium saucepan over medium heat.
8. Then, add onion and garlic and cook until soft and fragrant, about 7 minutes.
9. In the meantime, in a small bowl or measuring cup, whisk together milk, flour and garlic powder.
10. At this point, pour milk mixture into saucepan with the onions and garlic.
11. This is when you allow sauce to simmer, whisking continuously until sauce has thickened, about 5 minutes.
12. In addition, remove from heat and whisk in 2 cups shredded cheddar cheese until melted.
13. After that, pour cheese sauce over quinoa and broccoli. Toss well to combine.
14. Then, transfer to greased baking dish and top with remaining shredded cheese.
15. Finally, bake uncovered for about 15 minutes or until the casserole is heated through and cheese has melted.
16. Serve warm.

Naan Pizza with Butternut Squash and Pesto

Prep Time: 10 minutes

Cook Time: 45 minutes

Yield: 3

Tip:

This recipe topped with roasted butternut squash, pesto and gouda cheese makes for an easy vegetarian weeknight meal or better still an impressive party appetizer.

Ingredients

Naan Pizza

> 1 (about 14.5 ounce) can fire roasted diced tomatoes, drained
>
> ½ cup of grated Parmesan cheese
>
> 1–2 Tablespoons of fresh basil (for garnish)
>
> ½ cup of shredded Gouda cheese
>
> ¼ cup of pesto (use recipe below)
>
> 3 pieces of garlic naan

Butternut Squash

> 1 ½ teaspoons of olive oil
>
> sea salt
>
> 2 cups of peeled and chopped butternut squash (about ¼ – ½ inch cubes)

Pesto

> 1 clove of garlic
>
> 2 Tablespoons of olive oil
>
> 1 cup of fresh basil leaves
>
> 2 Tablespoons of pine nuts

½ cup of grated parmesan

Directions:

    a. Meanwhile, heat oven to 400°F.
    b. After which you spread chopped butternut squash on a baking dish.
    c. After that, toss with 1 teaspoon oil and sprinkle with sea salt.
    d. Then, bake for 20-25 minutes or until squash is tender.

2. Furthermore, while squash is roasting, make pesto by blending together garlic, parmesan, basil, pine nuts and olive oil until relatively smooth.
3. After which you place 3 pieces of naan bread on a baking sheet.
4. At this point, sprinkle gouda over naan, leaving a 1/4-inch border.
5. This is when you top with roasted squash and diced tomatoes.
6. In addition, using a teaspoon, drop pesto over naan pizzas. Sprinkle each with parmesan.
7. After that, bake at 400°F for 20 minutes or until edges of the naan are lightly browned and cheese has melted.
8. Finally, top with fresh basil and serve.

Butternut Squash Fries

Prep Time: 10 minutes

Cook Time: 40 minutes

Yield: 4

Ingredients

sea salt

1 butternut squash (about 4 cups)

Directions:

1. Meanwhile, heat oven to 425°F.
2. After which you peel the squash. (optional)
3. After that, cut the butternut squash in half and de-seed it like you would a cantaloupe.
4. Then, cut it up into French fry shapes. NOTE: try to make the pieces similar in size so that they finish cooking at the same time.
5. At this point, place on a baking sheet lined with parchment paper or sprayed with nonstick cooking spray.
6. This is when you sprinkle lightly with sea salt.
7. Furthermore, place tray in your pre-heated oven and bake for 40 minutes or so, flipping halfway through baking process.
8. Remember, fries are done when they are starting to brown a little.
9. Finally, serve with ketchup or your favorite French fry dipping sauce.

Goat Cheese Stuffed Dates

Prep Time: 15 minutes

Cook Time: 10 minutes

Yield: 34

Tip:

However, these sweet and savory goat cheese stuffed dates topped with roasted pecans and fresh thyme are a quick and easy appetizer that everyone will love.

Ingredients

4 oz. of goat cheese

1 Tablespoon of maple syrup

1/8 teaspoon of sea salt

17 medjool dates

½ cup of pecan halves

1 teaspoon of fresh thyme + more for garnish

1/8 teaspoon of paprika

Directions:

1. Meanwhile, heat oven to 400°F.
2. After which you chop pecans and add to a small bowl with paprika, maple syrup, salt and fresh thyme.
3. After that, toss pecans and spread on a baking sheet lined with parchment.
4. Then, roast pecans for about 8-10 minutes; remove from oven and let cool.
5. At this point, cut dates in half and remove pit.
6. Finally, stuff each date with goat cheese, top with pecans and garnish with fresh thyme.

Mediterranean Salmon Salad

Prep Time: 10 mins

Cook Time: 12 mins

Yield: 1

Tip:

This recipe is loaded with flavor, incredibly healthy and gluten-free.

Ingredients

Salmon

- 1 teaspoon of olive oil
- Sea salt and pepper (I prefer this Piquant Spice Grinder)
- 1 (4 oz.) piece of salmon
- 1 teaspoon of lemon juice

Salad

- 1 head romaine lettuce (chopped)
- ¼ cup of cooked quinoa
- ¼ cup of red onion (chopped)
- ¼ cup of grape tomatoes (chopped)
- 2 Tablespoons of feta cheese
- 1 Tablespoon of chopped almonds

Dressing

- 1 Tablespoon of fresh lemon juice
- Sea salt and pepper (to taste)
- 1 Tablespoon of olive oil
- ½ teaspoon of Dijon mustard
- ½ teaspoon of maple syrup or honey (optional)

Directions:

1. Meanwhile, heat oven to 400°F.
2. After which you rub the salmon with olive oil and season both sides with salt and pepper.
3. After that, place fillet skin-side down on a baking sheet, pour the lemon juice over top and roast for 10-12 minutes or until just cooked through. (NOTE: time will vary based on the size of your salmon; watch it carefully as you don't want to overcook it).
4. Then, while salmon is cooking, make dressing by whisking together all the ingredients.
5. Furthermore, prep salad by adding chopped romaine to a large salad bowl, and top with quinoa, tomatoes, red onion, feta cheese and chopped almonds.
6. Finally, once salmon is cooked through, remove from oven and place it on top of salad.
7. Then, drizzle dressing over salad and enjoy.

Asian Tofu Tacos

Prep Time: 20 minutes

Cook Time: 20 minutes

Yield: 4

Tips:

1. Make sure you spice up Taco Tuesday with these flavorful and meatless Asian tofu tacos.
2. Remember, the tofu is crispy and flavorful and pairs great with the crunchy and refreshing slaw.

Ingredients

3 Tablespoons of low-sodium soy sauce or tamari

2 teaspoons of garlic powder

hoisin sauce (for serving)

1 lb. of extra firm tofu, pressed and chopped into ½ inch cubes

1 Tablespoon of sesame oil

Asian slaw

4–8 flour or corn tortillas (depending on size)

Directions:

1. **Meanwhile,** heat oven to 400°F.
2. After which you prep tofu and prepare sauce by combining tamari, sesame oil and garlic powder in a large bowl.
3. After that, you toss tofu in sauce.
4. Then, add to a rimmed baking sheet and bake tofu for about 20 minutes, flipping around the 10-minute mark.
5. At this point, tofu should be golden and slightly crisp.
6. Furthermore, while tofu is baking, make Asian slaw recipe.
7. Finally, once tofu is done, prep tacos by adding a portion of tofu and slaw into each tortilla.
8. You can serve with lime wedges and hoisin sauce for drizzling on top.

Asian Slaw

Prep Time: 20 minutes

Total Time: 20 minutes

Yield: 8

Tips:

This recipe is a quick and easy Asian slaw loaded with crunchy vegetables and tossed in a flavorful Asian dressing.

It is perfect as a topping for tacos or as a side!

Ingredients

Slaw

- 1 cup of shredded carrots
- white or black sesame seeds (for topping)
- 1 lb. (about 5 cups) shredded cabbage
- 1 cup of sliced scallions
- 1 red bell pepper, thinly sliced (about 1 cup)

Asian Dressing

- 3 Tablespoons of mayonnaise (I prefer avocado oil mayo, but vegan mayo works too)
- 2 Tablespoons of low-sodium tamari (coconut aminos or better still soy sauce works too)
- 1 Tablespoon of mirin
- 1 tablespoon of grated ginger
- 2 Tablespoons of sesame oil (I prefer spicy sesame oil)
- 1 Tablespoon of rice vinegar

Directions:

1. First, toss together slaw ingredients in a large salad bowl.
2. After which you add all ingredients for the dressing into a blender and blend until smooth and creamy.
3. After that, pour over slaw and toss to combine.
4. Finally, top with sesame seeds and serve.
5. Remember, slaw will keep for 4-5 days in the fridge.

Notes

   a. However, for the cabbage, you can use Napa, green or red.
   b. For me, I prefer a combo of green and red for extra color.

Baked Peanut Tofu

Prep Time: 1 hour 15 minutes

Cook Time: 30 minutes

Yield: 4

Tips:

This recipe is marinated in a delicious peanut sauce that gives the tofu an amazing flavor and crispy coating.

All you do is just pair with rice and a veggie side for a full meal!

Ingredients

If you want to serve: rice of choice and veggies

1 (16oz) package of extra-firm tofu, pressed to remove liquid

Peanut Sauce

1/8 cup of hot water

2 Tablespoons of rice vinegar

¼ teaspoon of red pepper flakes (add more for more spice)

¼ cup of peanut butter

1 Tablespoon of tamari (or soy sauce)

1 Tablespoon of miso paste

Directions:

1. First, once tofu has been pressed, chop into ½ inch cubes.
2. After which you add rice vinegar, water, tamari, peanut butter, miso paste and red pepper flakes into a bowl and whisk until smooth. NOTE: you can also use a blender for this.
3. After that, pour the sauce over the tofu cubes and toss to cover all the pieces.
4. Then, marinate the tofu in peanut sauce and place in a covered container in the fridge for at least an hour. NOTE: I marinated mine for about 5-6 hours.
5. Meanwhile, heat oven to 350°F.

6. At this point, place marinated tofu on a baking sheet sprayed with cooking spray and bake for about 30-40 minutes, flipping once around the 15-minute mark.
7. Finally, remove from oven and serve tofu with sides of choice. **NOTE:** I like to serve it with rice and some sort of veggie and I also like adding a little Sriracha on top for extra heat.

Butternut Tofu Sheet Pan Dinner

Prep Time: 20 minutes

Cook Time: 70 minutes

Yield: 4

Tip:

1. This recipe features tofu, butternut squash, chickpeas, and red onion.
2. However, everything is roasted and served with a creamy tahini sauce for a flavorful, protein-packed meal.

Ingredients

2 Tablespoons of liquid aminos, coconut aminos or low-sodium tamari

½ teaspoon of garlic powder

1 (15-ounce) can chickpeas, drained and rinsed

2 Tablespoons of olive or better still avocado oil

½ teaspoon of ground pepper

¼ cup of coarsely chopped cilantro leaves, for garnish

1 lb. extra-firm tofu, pressed, drained and chopped into 1-inch pieces

1 Tablespoon of maple syrup

1 medium butternut squash (about 6 cups) peeled, seeded and cut into 1-inch pieces

1 medium/large red onion (roughly chopped)

½ teaspoon of sea salt

tahini sauce

Directions:

1. First, add chopped tofu, maple syrup, aminos, and garlic powder in a large bowl.
2. After which you toss and let marinate for at least 30 minutes.

3. After that, prep tahini sauce while tofu is marinating.
4. Meanwhile, heat oven to 375°F.
5. At this point, add chopped butternut squash, chickpeas, and onion to a large sheet pan.
6. Then, drizzle on the oil, sprinkle with salt and pepper and toss to coat.
7. This is when you add tofu to the pan and toss once more.
8. Furthermore, place sheet pan in the oven and roast for about 30 minutes, toss ingredients and place bake in the oven for about 40 minutes or until chickpeas are crisp, tofu is golden and butternut squash is fork-tender.
9. Finally, portion butternut squash, chickpea, tofu mixture onto plates, garnish with cilantro and drizzle with tahini sauce.
10. You can serve with extra tahini sauce.

Baked Sweet Potato Fries

Prep Time: 10 minutes

Cook Time: 40 minutes

Yield: 4

Tips:

This recipe will make you satisfy your craving for fries with healthy baked sweet potato fries that are actually crispy!

It is perfect for serving alongside a burger or sandwich.

Ingredients

2 Tablespoons of avocado (or better still olive oil)

½ teaspoon of garlic powder

sea salt, to taste (added after baking)

2 medium – large sweet potato, cut into thin slices (about ¼ inch)

1 Tablespoon of arrowroot powder (or better still cornstarch)

½ teaspoon of pepper

Directions:

1. Meanwhile, heat oven to 425°F and line a large baking sheet (affiliate link) with parchment.
2. After which you place sweet potato slices into a large bowl and toss with oil, arrowroot powder, garlic powder and pepper.
3. After that, spread the fries onto your prepared baking sheet, making sure the fries aren't crowded. NOTE: you may find that you need to use two baking sheets.
4. Remember, the fries can't be crowded or else they will start to steam and get soft rather than crispy.
5. At this point, bake for 15 minutes, take them out of the oven and flip, then bake for another 15-20 minutes.
6. Finally, keep an eye on them the last 5 minutes as some of the smaller pieces might start to burn.

One Pan Roasted Veggie and Chicken Sausage

Prep Time: 10 minutes

Cook Time: 25 minutes

Yield: 4

Tips:

Sweet potatoes, broccoli and red onion come together with chicken sausage for a simple, healthy sheet pan meal that's delicious and perfect for busy weeknights.

Ingredients

- 2 crowns broccoli (chopped into bite-size florets)
- 1 red onion (peeled and roughly chopped)
- ½ teaspoon of sea salt
- 2 Tablespoons of olive oil (or better still avocado oil)
- Quinoa, rice, or whole grain, for serving (optional)
- 5 organic chicken sausage links (any flavor), chopped into bite-size chunks
- 2 sweet potatoes (chopped into bite-size chunks)
- 3 cloves garlic (minced)
- ½ teaspoon of ground pepper
- Sriracha, for topping (it is optional)

Directions:

1. Meanwhile, heat oven to 400°F.
2. After which you chop everything and then toss your broccoli, onion, sausage, sweet potato chunks, and garlic on the baking sheet.
3. After that, drizzle oil over sausage and veggie mixture, sprinkle on salt and pepper and toss to combine.

4. Then, place the baking sheet in the pre-heated oven and bake for 15 minutes.
5. At this point, toss the mixture using a spatula and bake for another 10-15 minutes or until sweet potatoes are fork-tender.
6. Finally, season with additional salt and pepper, to taste and serve over cooked rice or quinoa with sriracha sauce, if using.

Pear Salad with Walnuts, Avocado and Grilled Chicken

Prep Time: 20 minutes

Yield: 2

Tip:

However, this combo makes for a satisfying meal-sized salad that's perfect for pear season!

Ingredients

2 pears (I prefer Red Anjou and Green Bartlett), sliced or chopped

2 slices of cooked turkey bacon

2 Tablespoons of dried cranberries

½ avocado, sliced or better still chopped into chunks

6 cups of spring mix

6 oz. of grilled chicken breast

¼ cup of goat cheese crumbles

2 Tablespoons of chopped walnuts (raw or toasted)

Maple Balsamic Dressing

¼ cup of olive oil

1 teaspoon of Dijon mustard

¼ teaspoon of Italian seasoning

½ cup of balsamic vinegar (I prefer white)

1 teaspoon of maple syrup

1 teaspoon of minced garlic

½ teaspoon of sea salt

Directions:

1. First, cook turkey bacon and grill chicken if you haven't already.
2. After which you prepare dressing by whisking together all ingredients in a small bowl or jar. NOTE: I prefer using a jar with a lid for this so you can easily store any leftover dressing in the fridge in that same jar.

Direction to prep salad:

1. **First, g**rab two bowls and add a base of spring mix, grilled chicken breast, bacon, goat cheese, pear slices, dried cranberries, walnuts and avocado.
2. Finally, drizzle salad with desired amount of balsamic dressing and enjoy!

Healthy Sweet Potato Fries Recipe

Tip:

This savory recipe baked with coconut oil, garlic, salt, basil, and other spices.

Course Side

Prep Time 10 minutes

Cook Time 30 minutes

Servings 4 +

Ingredients

- Spices of choice such as garlic sea salt, basil, pepper, oregano, and thyme
- 2-3 large sweet potatoes
- ¼ cup of olive oil (or melted coconut oil)

Directions:

1. Meanwhile, heat oven to 400°F.
2. After which you mix olive oil and spices together in a small bowl.
3. After that, slice sweet potatoes into desired size and put on large baking sheet (or two if you are making a lot).
4. Then, pour the oil/seasoning mixture over the fries and toss by hand until evenly coated.
5. Finally, bake for about 25-30 minutes or more until slightly browned and tender.
6. You can serve with homemade ketchup or mayo (It is a French thing!).

Notes

Feel free to play with the spices to suit your tastes - lemon pepper, Cajun, cinnamon and spice?

Healthy Onion Rings Recipe

Tip:

This recipe is a healthy homemade onion rings that are grain free!

Course Side

Prep Time 5 minutes

Cook Time 10 minutes

Servings 2 servings

Ingredients

- ½ cup of coconut flour
- ½ teaspoon of garlic powder
- ½ teaspoon of pepper
- 1 large onion
- tallow lard (or coconut oil)
- ¼ cup of arrowroot (or tapioca powder)
- 1 teaspoon of salt
- 2 eggs melted butter (or coconut milk)

Directions:

1. First, heat fat (lard, tallow, or coconut oil) over medium-high heat in a large, deep, skillet or deep fryer (preferable).
2. After which you mix coconut flour, arrowroot, and spices on a large plate.
3. After that, beat eggs in a bowl or put melted butter or milk in a bowl.
4. Then, peel and thinly slice whole onion into rings.
5. At this point, separate rings and dip into egg mixture (or substitute), then into coconut mixture.
6. Furthermore, drop into hot oil and cook about 3 minutes per side until golden brown and crispy.

7. Finally, remove, let cool, and enjoy.

NOTE:

1. I like to salt the rings after cooking.
2. Remember, the arrowroot powder is needed to help the coconut flour stick to the onion rings.

Shrimp & Cucumber Appetizers

Tip:

This recipe is a fresh and light appetizer of shrimp on top of cucumber slices with cream cheese.

Course Appetizer

Prep Time 5 minutes

Cook Time 5 minutes

Servings 2 -4

Ingredients

- ½ cup of strained Greek yogurt (or better still cream cheese)
- 12 precooked shrimp
- 1 cucumber
- 1 teaspoon of dried or fresh dill (optional)
- Pinch of sea salt and sprinkle of pepper

Directions:

1. First, peel the cucumber in alternating strips to leave a striped look on the outside.
2. After which you slice the cucumber into ¼ to ½ inch slices and put on a plate.
3. After that, mix the strained Greek yogurt or cream cheese with the dill, salt, and pepper.
4. Then, put a small amount of the yogurt mix on top of each piece of cucumber and top each one with a shrimp.
5. Finally, serve immediately or keep in the refrigerator for up to six hours.

Notes

1. However, strain yogurt by placing it in a cheesecloth or towel over a bowl for a few hours and use the part left in the towel.
2. Feel free to also use cream cheese, but this version has probiotics.

Easy Zucchini Fritters Recipe

Tip:

This recipe is easy to make and a great alternative to hash browns and tater tots with an extra nutrient boost!

Course Side

Prep Time 10 minutes

Cook Time 20 minutes

Servings 16 fritters

Ingredients

- 1 teaspoon of salt
- 2 eggs
- ¼ cup of almond flour
- 1 teaspoon of basil leaf
- 2 medium fresh zucchini (or better still 1½ cups frozen shredded zucchini, thawed)
- 1 small onion
- ½ cup of Parmesan cheese (or better still almond flour, or 3 Tablespoons of coconut flour)
- 1 teaspoon of garlic powder
- 1 teaspoon of black pepper

Directions:

1. Meanwhile, heat oven to 400°F.
2. After which you grease a baking sheet or muffin tin.
3. After that, grate the zucchini with a box grater or food processor.
4. Then, add the salt and squeeze very tightly with a towel to get the excess liquid out.

5. At this point, put in a medium sized bowl.
6. This is when you grate the onion and add to the bowl.
7. Furthermore, add the eggs, almond flour, Parmesan cheese, and spices and mix until combined.
8. After that, put Tablespoon size amounts of the mixture onto the baking sheet or fill the muffin tins ½ full.
9. In addition, bake for approximately 18-20 minutes or until tops and sides are starting to brown.
10. Finally, serve alone or with homemade ketchup. (NOTE: can also pan fry in coconut oil for a crispier outer coating).
11. Enjoy!

Notes

You can store in the refrigerator or freezer.

Healthy Chocolate Chip Cookies Recipe

Tips: in this recipe you can make a double batch and freeze the dough for later use.

However, you can either freeze in a tub or roll into balls and freeze in a single-layer on a parchment paper lined baking sheet.

Finally, once frozen store cookie dough balls in a bag or bucket in freezer until ready to use.

Course Dessert

Prep Time 10 minutes

Cook Time 20 minutes

Servings 24 cookies

Ingredients

- 2 cups of almond flour
- ½ teaspoon of baking soda
- ¼ to 1/3 cup of cane sugar
- Pinch of salt
- ½ cup of butter (or better still coconut oil softened)
- 1 large egg
- 1 Tablespoon of vanilla extract
- 1 cup of organic dark chocolate chips

Directions:

1. Meanwhile, heat the oven to 350°F.
2. After which you mix together the baking soda, almond flour, sugar, and salt in a bowl.
3. After that, add the softened butter or coconut oil (or a mix of both) and stir well by hand until mixed. **NOTE:** It should form a thick dough that is hard to stir.

4. Then, add the egg and vanilla and mix well. **NOTE:** this should make the dough easier to mix. Remember, if needed, add a teaspoon or two of milk or water to thin.
5. At this point, finished dough should be easy to form.
6. This is when you add chocolate chips and stir by hand until incorporated.
7. Furthermore, form dough into tablespoon size balls and bake for 10 minutes or until tops are starting to brown (NOTE: the centers will be somewhat soft, but they will firm up a bit as they cool).
8. Finally, let cool at least 5 minutes and serve.
9. Enjoy!

Chia Seed Energy Bars Recipe

Tip:

This is a delicious chia seed energy bars with coconut oil and dates for a natural energy boost.

Course Breakfast

Prep Time 20 minutes

Servings 4 bars

Ingredients

- ½ cup of chia seeds
- ½ teaspoon of vanilla extract (optional)
- 2 Tablespoons of add ins optional: dark chocolate chips, shredded coconut, dried fruit
- 6 large Medjool dates
- 2 Tablespoons of coconut oil
- a pinch of ground cinnamon (optional)

Directions:

1. First, remove the pits from the dates and discard.
2. After which you pulse the dates in a food processor or blender until they form a paste.
3. After that, in a medium bowl, mix the date paste with the chia seeds, coconut oil, and any optional ingredients. **NOTE:** it will form a thick dough.
4. Then, roll this dough into balls or press into the bottom of a glass or silicon baking dish and cut into squares.
5. This recipe can be eaten immediately in dough-form. I prefer to put it in the refrigerator or freezer to give it more of a chewy texture.

Notes

You can use an alternate dried fruit such as raisins, prunes, or apricots to form the paste.

For additional calcium, I suggest you add about a teaspoon of eggshell powder!

Snacks

Chocolate Coconut Energy Bars Recipe

Tip:

An easy, healthy, grain-free energy bar made with coconut, chocolate, and honey for an energy-boosting snack.

Course Snack

Prep Time 5 minutes

Cook Time 5 minutes

Servings 12 bars

Ingredients

- ½ cup of coconut oil
- ½ cup of cocoa powder
- ½ cup of chia seeds (or better still additional coconut)
- stevia tincture for extra sweetness (optional)
- ½ cup of cocoa butter
- ¼ cup of honey or to taste
- 1½ cups of shredded coconut unsweetened
- 1 teaspoon of vanilla extract (optional)

Directions:

1. First, melt the cocoa butter in a small pan over low heat.
2. After which you add coconut oil and melt.
3. After that, add honey and stir well.
4. Then, stir in cocoa powder.
5. At this point, stir in the shredded coconut and chia seeds.
6. This is when you add vanilla and stevia tincture if using.
7. Furthermore, pour into a parchment paper lined 9x13 baking dish and refrigerate for 1 hour or until hardened (can also freeze).

8. Finally, cut into squares/bars and enjoy!

Notes

I don't suggest you eating these in the evening! REASON: They tend to give a little too much energy!

Kale Chips Recipe

Course Snack

Prep Time 5 minutes

Cook Time 5 minutes

Servings 12 leaves

Ingredients

- 2 Tablespoons of olive oil
- ¼ teaspoon of sea salt
- 1 bunch kale (about 12 leaves)

Directions:

1. Meanwhile, heat to oven to 370°F.
2. After which you make sure kale leaves are washed and dried well.
3. After that, remove stems. (**NOTE:** this is optional; I actually often leave them in and just eat the leaves off of the stems).
4. Then, brush or rub the leaves with olive oil until well coated and sprinkle with sea salt to taste.
5. At this point, place the leaves in a single layer on a large baking sheet.
6. Furthermore, place in the preheated oven for 5-10 minutes or less. NOTE: you will need to watch them closely and remove them as soon as they are crispy and barely browning.
7. Finally, serve immediately or leave uncovered on the counter on a plate for up to 3 days.

Notes

You should try adding spices like cumin and chili powder or ginger and garlic for a different taste.

If your leftover kale chips get soggy, I suggest you toss them back in the oven for a few minutes to re-crisp them.

Snow Cream Recipe

Course Snack

Prep Time 5 minutes

Total Time 5 minutes

Servings 4

Ingredients

- 1 cup or more of coconut milk or better still raw milk
- honey or maple syrup to taste (it is optional)
- fresh clean snow
- ½ teaspoon of vanilla extract

Directions:

1. First, collect a large amount of fresh snow in a large bowl.
2. After which in a smaller bowl, combine some of the snow, vanilla, and any desired sweetener.
3. After that, add just enough coconut milk or milk to create a smooth consistency.
4. Then, mix well with a spoon until evenly mixed.
5. Finally, serve immediately and enjoy.

Notes

However, snow cream must be eaten immediately as it loses its consistency if kept in the freezer.

Homemade Fruit Snacks Recipe

This is a healthy homemade fruit snacks packed with nutrients from gelatin, fruit, kombucha (optional), and juice.

Course Snack

Prep Time 5 minutes

Cook Time 10 minutes

Servings 24 +

Ingredients

- ¼ cup of honey or maple syrup (optional)
- 8 Tablespoons of gelatin powder
- 2 cups of fruit juice OR kombucha OR some other liquid of choice
- 1 cup of berries pureed (it is optional)

Directions:

1. First, combine fruit juice or kombucha and honey/maple syrup if using in a small saucepan.
2. After which you heat over low heat until warm and starting to simmer, but not hot or boiling.
3. After that, add pureed fruit, if using.
4. Then, sprinkle the gelatin over the juice mixture while whisking or using an immersion blender.
5. At this point, continue doing this until all gelatin is incorporated and the mixture is smooth.
6. Furthermore, adding the gelatin too quickly will make it more difficult to get the mixture to incorporate. NOTE: an immersion blender is not necessary but greatly speeds up the process.
7. Finally, as soon as the gelatin is mixed in and the mixture is smooth, pour into molds or a lined/greased baking dish and place in the refrigerator or freezer until hardened.

Notes

It is essential to have all ingredients ready before beginning as you'll need to work quickly once you start the process.

However, make sure you are using gelatin, not collagen hydrolysate or peptides as they will not gel. Remember, the Great Lakes brand of gelatin doesn't work well in this recipe.

Lactation Cookies Recipe (Gluten Free)

These cookies are delicious and can be made ahead and put into the freezer.

Course Snack

Prep Time 10 minutes

Cook Time 36 minutes

Servings 4 dozen

Ingredients

- 1 tablespoon of anise seeds
- 1 cup of almonds soaked overnight and dehydrated
- ½ cup of coconut oil melted
- 1 cup of oatmeal soaked overnight
- 1 tablespoon of vanilla extract
- 5 eggs
- 1 cup of chocolate chips
- 2 Tablespoons of fenugreek seeds
- 1/3 cup of flax seeds
- 1 cup of mix of dates and prunes
- 1/3 cup of shredded coconut
- 1 cup of almond flour
- 1 teaspoon of baking powder
- ½ cup of honey or maple syrup (optional)

Directions:

1. Meanwhile, heat oven to 350°F.
2. After which you put fenugreek, anise and flax seeds, dates, almonds, and prunes into a food processor.
3. After which you blend until smooth.

4. Then, in a large bowl, mix together all remaining ingredients.
5. At this point, mix in date mixture until well combined.
6. Furthermore, spoon by heaping tablespoon onto a cookie sheet.
7. Finally, bake for 12 minutes.

Notes

Make sure you store in a sealed container at room temperature or freeze.

Feel free to freeze balls of cookie dough and then thaw and bake, or freeze them already baked!

Radish Cream Cheese Dip Recipe

However, this smooth and creamy dip is bursting with fresh flavor from the herbs and a hint of heat from the radishes.

Course Snack

Prep Time 5 minutes

Servings 3 cups

Ingredients

- 8 oz. cream cheese
- A handful of fresh parsley
- 1 bunch of radishes
- 1 cup of cottage cheese
- 5 fresh basil leaves

Directions:

1. First, wash the radishes well and cut off the tops and bottoms.
2. After which you add all ingredients to a food processor and puree until smooth.
3. Then, serve with veggies for dipping.

Smoked Salmon Dip Recipe

Tip:
This delicious savory salmon dip with dill and cottage cheese for extra protein and also a great appetizer or party snack or wonderful as a quick lunch.

Course Snack

Servings 2 cups

Ingredients

- ¼ cup of cream cheese
- 2 tablespoons of fresh dill (finely chopped)
- 1 teaspoon of lemon juice
- ½ teaspoon of smoked paprika
- 1 cup of cottage cheese
- 8 oz. smoked salmon (chopped)
- ¼ cup of green onion (finely sliced)
- 1 teaspoon of hot sauce (optional)

Directions:
1. First, put cottage cheese and cream cheese in a food processor and blend until smooth.
2. After which you add dill, smoked salmon, green onion, lemon juice, and hot sauce and mix by hand.
3. Then, spoon into serving dish and top with smoked paprika.

Notes
I bet you will enjoy this creamy dip on gluten-free crackers, with cucumber slices and carrot sticks, mixed into eggs, or on a bed of leafy greens.

Strawberry Fruit Leather Recipe (with Beets)

This recipe is a simple and nutrient-dense natural fruit leather snacks made with fresh strawberries, optional honey, and sneaky extra nutrients from beets.

Prep Time 5 minutes

Cook Time 3 hours

Servings 16 +

Ingredients

> 4 cups of fresh or frozen strawberries defrost if using frozen
>
> 2 Tablespoons of fresh lemon lime, or orange juice
>
> 2 medium beets peeled and steamed until soft (optional, use ½ cup extra strawberries if you don't use)
>
> ½ cup of honey or maple syrup (optional or ½ cup pitted dates)

Directions:

1. Meanwhile, heat the oven to 170°F or use a dehydrator.
2. After which you puree the cooled cooked beets, honey/maple syrup/dates, strawberries, and citrus juice in a blender until completely smooth.
3. After that, line two rimmed baking sheets with parchment paper or silicon baking mats (safe at low temperatures).
4. Then, pour/spread the mixture evenly onto the baking sheets.
5. At this point, place in oven and cook until firm and no longer sticky to the touch (3-4 hours in most ovens).
6. This is when you remove from oven and let cool.
7. Furthermore, cut into strips and roll up with parchment paper.
8. Finally, store in an air-tight container until ready to eat.

Notes

1. If you are using frozen defrosted berries, the liquid will be thinner but if using fresh berries, you may have to add a couple teaspoons of water to get the mixture smooth enough to spread.
2. Remember, the mixture should be pourable but not thin enough to run off the baking sheet.
3. This recipe can be stored in the refrigerator or freezer in an airtight container for up to a week (refrigerator) or two months (freezer).

DRINKS AND SMOOTHIES

Green Immunity Smoothie

Serves: 2

Ingredients

- ½ cup of water
- 1 small Lebanese cucumber
- 1 teaspoon of turmeric (**NOTE:** recipe calls for ½ teaspoons but you can go crazy with turmeric)
- Small handful of sprouts
- 1 cup of coconut water
- 1 cm piece ginger (peeled)
- 1 cup of spinach leaves
- juice of ½ lemon
- Optional: 1 cup of berries (NOTE: if using frozen berries, I suggest you allow them to thaw a bit)

Directions:

1. First, add everything to a blender and blitz until smooth.
2. After which you pour into jars.
3. After that, add berries and puree.
4. Then, divide equally between jars and give them a swirl.
5. Enjoy fresh.

Two seconds chia pudding smoothie

Serves one to go

Ingredients

> 1 frozen banana (pre-peeled and pre-cut into chunks)
>
> 1 ½ cups of already made chia pudding (I almost always use this Coconut chia pudding recipe)
>
> Optional: however, if you have anything else right next to your blender, ready to be used, feel free to add. I added a handful of dry blueberries to this smoothie (thus the purple hue) and sprinkled some granola.

Directions:

1. First, add all the ingredients to a blender, blitz for few seconds.
2. Finally, pour into a jar and get busy with your day, while enjoying a healthy breakfast on the way.

Almond fig and strawberry smoothie

Serves: 1

Ingredients

4 ripe figs (**NOTE:** you want organic because you're eating the skin too)

1 big frozen banana (cut into chunks)

Pinch of vanilla seeds

1 ½ cups almond milk (go homemade!)

A handful of ripe strawberries (**NOTE:** strawberries soak up A LOT of pesticides)

2 Tablespoons of chia seeds

Optional: A Medjool date / 2 regular dates if you prefer your smoothie on the sweeter side (**NOTE:** I find it sweet enough already)

Toppings as your heart desires

Directions:

First, add everything to a blender, whiz until smooth, enjoy and be happy.

Mango peach match a smoothie

Prep time: 2 mins

Serves: 1 big smoothie / 2 regular

Base ingredients:

    2 bananas

    1 mango

    1 teaspoon turmeric

    1 cup of water

    2 celery stalks (leaves included)

    1 peach

    1 Tablespoon of chia seeds

    juice of ½ a lemon

    1 cup of coconut water

To layer it up:

    ½ teaspoon spirulina

    ½ cup of hemp seeds / quinoa flakes / rolled oats

    ½ teaspoon of match a powder

    Optional toppings: blueberry lollies, pomegranate gems

Directions:

1. First, add the base ingredients to a blender and whiz until smooth.
2. After which you pour half the smoothie into one or two jars.
3. After that, add the match a and spirulina to the remaining smoothie in the blender and process for a few seconds.
4. Finally, gently sprinkle the hemp/quinoa/oats onto the first layer of the smoothie then pour the second layer.

Tip: best enjoyed right away with toppings of choice.

Matcha cranberry Christmas smoothie bowl

Prep time: 2 mins

Serves 1

Ingredients:

> 1 ripe peach (pitted)
>
> ¼ cup of hemp hearts (it is optional)
>
> 2 Tablespoons of flax meal
>
> Water to blend (about 1 to 1 ½ cups)
>
> 1 big banana or better still 2 smaller ones
>
> ½ cup of wholegrain oats
>
> 2 Tablespoons of chia seeds
>
> 1 Tablespoon of match a green tea
>
> **Toppings:** 2/3 cups of cranberries (fresh or frozen), coconut flakes, goji berries, poppy seeds

Directions:

1. First, add all the ingredients except toppings to a blender and whiz up until thick, creamy and smooth.
2. Then, scoop into a bowl, add toppings and enjoy.

Coconut dessert smoothie

Prep time: 1 min

Serves 1

Ingredients:

- 1 banana
- 1/3 cup of quinoa flakes
- 1 young coconut (water and flesh)
- 1 Tablespoon of maca powder
- Optional toppings: maple syrup & cacao nibs

Directions:

1. First, crack open your coconut.
2. After which you strain the water to make sure it doesn't have any impurities. **NOTE:** clean the flesh to make sure it doesn't have pieces of shell.
3. After that, add coconut water and meat to the blender with the rest of the ingredients and blitz.
4. Then, serve right away.

Tip: for best result, use a chilled young coconut.

Green fruits and basil smoothie

Prep time: 5 mins

Serves: 1-2

Ingredients:

- ½ cucumber
- 1 green apple
- 1 big banana
- 1 Tablespoon of chia seeds
- 1 cup of basil
- 1 celery rib
- 1 pear
- 1 piece of ginger (**NOTE:** however big/small you fancy, depending how much you love ginger)
- 1 Tablespoon tahini
- Remember to add enough water to blend. Start with 1 ½ cups and continue to add ½ cup at a time, as needed.
- Optional: 1 teaspoon of match a green tea
- Optional to serve: as a smoothie bowl, I suggest you topped with granola

Directions:

First, chuck everything to blender, blitz and serve right away.

NOTE: this smoothie oxidizes quite fast because of the basil.

Banana 'n berries quinoa smoothie

Prep time: 5 mins

Serves: 1-2

Ingredients

For the orange layer: 1 blood orange, 1/3 cup of sesame seeds, 2 bananas, ½ cup of quinoa flakes, ¼ cup of filtered water, ½ cup puffed quinoa.

For the berry layer: 2/3 cups mixed frozen berries, 2 Tablespoons of chia seeds, 1 banana, juice of 1 lemon, ¼ cup filtered water.

To serve: 4 lemon ice cubes

Directions:

1. First, add all the ingredients for the orange layer to the blender and whiz.
2. After which you pour into a big mason jar or 2 smaller individual jars or glasses.
3. After that, add the ingredients for the berry layer to the blender (no need to wash it) and whiz.
4. Then, scoop the puffed quinoa on top of the orange layer then pour the berry smoothie mix on top.
5. Finally, drop some lemon ice cubes and serve right away; in the sunshine.

Celery apple berry smoothie

Prep time: 5 mins

Serves: 1-2

Ingredients

- 1 big seasonal apple
- juice of 1 lime
- 1 cup of mixed berries
- 1-2 cups of water, start with 1 cup and only add more if needed to reach your desired consistency
- 2 celery ribs
- 2 ginger (slices)
- 1 frozen banana (cubed)

Directions:

First, add all to blender and whiz away.

It can be best enjoyed fresh. (**NOTE:** but keeps overnight).

Golden Smoothie to mark a golden milestone

Prep time: 5 mins

Serves: 1

Ingredients

- big handful of mango (NOTE: you can use fresh or frozen)
- 1 cup of water
- 1/3 cup of hemp seeds
- 1 small frozen banana (cut into chunks)
- 1 Tablespoon of maca powder
- Optional topping: raw bee pollen

Directions:

1. First, add all to blender and whiz.
2. Enjoy fresh!

Notes

However, this smoothie is not overly sweet.

You can add a tablespoon of your favorite sweetener, if you want.

Masala chai iced coconut drink

Prep time: 5 mins

Serves: 1-2

Ingredients

- 3 cups of water
- 6 whole cloves
- 1/3 teaspoon of ground cinnamon
- Seeds of 2 green cardamom pods (crushed)
- 1 Tablespoon of sweetener of choice (raw honey, maple syrup) + 2 Tablespoons of warm water
- Water and meat of one young coconut
- 1 teaspoon of thin ginger slices
- 2-star anise
- Pinch of freshly ground nutmeg
- good pinch of fennel seeds (crushed)
- Optional: 2 teabags of your favorite chai or better still about 4-5 teaspoons of loose leaf chai (**NOTE:** you can also leave it out and make a caffeine free drink – absolutely gorgeous on its own too!)

Directions:

1. First, add the coconut meat, coconut water and 3 cups of water to the blender and whiz on high speed until creamy and smooth.
2. After which you pour in a mason jar and add ginger, star anise, cloves, cinnamon and nutmeg.
3. After that, crush cardamom and fennel seeds with a mortar and pestle and add them to the drink.
4. Then, mix sweetener with a couple of tablespoons of warm water until dissolved.
5. At this point, add to the drink and add the chai too, if using.
6. This is when you put the lid on the mason jar, give it a good shake and place it in the fridge.

7. Furthermore, allow it to cold brew overnight or for at least 12 hours.
8. Finally, strain the drink with a regular sieve or nut milk bag and serve chilled with a dash of cinnamon and with ice, if you prefer.

Cold brewed French Earl Grey iced tea

Serves: 1 L

Ingredients

- 550 ml water
- 1 teaspoon of sweetener of choice (honey / maple syrup) + 2 Tablespoons warm water
- Water of 1 young coconut (**NOTE:** I got about 450 ml)
- 3 teaspoons of Deitea French Earl Grey loose leaf

Directions:

1. First, mix the honey or maple syrup with the warm water to help dissolve it.
2. After which you combine honey, tea, coconut water and water in a mason jar, pop the lid and place it in the fridge.
3. After that, let it brew overnight.
4. Then, strain and serve the next day with orange slices or fresh mint.

Green bliss greens smoothie with mango and peach

Prep time: 5 mins

Serves: 1-2

Ingredients

- 1 big kale leaf
- 1 big frozen banana
- 1 peach
- 1 cup of extra water or as needed
- Water and meat from 1 young coconut
- 1 celery rib
- 1 mango (or heap handful of frozen mango)
- 1 teaspoon of match a
- **Serve:** you can serve with chia seeds and fresh mint
- **Optional:** ice cubes

Directions:

First, chuck everything to a blender, whiz it up, add toppings and enjoy fresh.

Cold brewed French Earl Grey iced tea

Serves: 1 L

Ingredients

- 550 ml water
- 1 teaspoon sweetener of choice (honey / maple syrup) + 2 Tablespoons of warm water
- Water of 1 young coconut (**NOTE:** I got about 450 ml)
- 3 teaspoons of Deitea French Earl Grey loose leaf

Directions:

1. First, mix the honey or maple syrup with the warm water to help dissolve it.
2. After which you combine tea, honey, coconut water and water in a mason jar, pop the lid and place it in the fridge.
3. After that, let it brew overnight.
4. Finally, strain and serve the next day with orange slices or fresh mint.

The perfect summer smoothie

Prep time: 5 mins

Serves: 1-2

Ingredients

- 1 big apple (**NOTE:** go for what's in season)
- Handful of strawberries
- 1 cup of coconut water
- About 10 cups cooled watermelon cubes
- 1 banana
- Handful of mint
- Optional: toppings of choice

Directions:

1. First, chuck all to blender and whiz it up.
2. Make sure you enjoy fresh.

Delicious afternoon picks me up: coconut berry smoothie

Prep time: 5 mins

Serves: 1-2

Ingredients

- 2 celery ribs
- A handful of cucumber slices/chunks
- More water, if needed (**NOTE:** depending on how much water you get from your coconut)
- Water of 1 young green coconut (chilled)
- 1 frozen banana
- Two handfuls of berries of choice (**NOTE:** I used currants, blackberries, raspberries and strawberries)
- 1 cup of melon chunks

Directions:

First, add all to blender and whiz it up.

It is best served right away, chilled.

Lettuce be healthy breakfast smoothie

Cook time: 5 mins

Serves: 1-2

Ingredients

- 1 small ripe avocado
- 8 loquats (or 2 apricots / 1 peach / 1/2 mango)
- 2 Tablespoons of sesame seeds
- ½ teaspoon to 1 teaspoon of match a green tea
- 5 lemon juice frozen ice cubes (or better still ¼ cup lemon juice + ice cubes)
- Handful of shredded lettuce
- 1 banana
- flesh of 1 big juicy orange
- handful of fresh mint leaves
- 1 teaspoon of bee pollen (optional)

If you want to serve: chia seeds, pumpkin seeds and fresh mint leaves

Directions:

First, add all to blender and whiz until smooth.

Apple rosemary and cinnamon ice tea

Makes 2 L

Ingredients

- 1 cinnamon stick
- 2 L boiling water
- 1 whole red apple (cored, thinly sliced)
- 1 rosemary sprig

If you want to serve: ice, fresh apple slices, fresh seasonal fruits (NOTE: I prefer cherries and limes, but oranges or mandarins would be beautiful too)

Directions:

1. First, add sliced apple, cinnamon and rosemary to a glass bowl or a pot.
2. After which you add 2 liters of boiling water, stir a couple of times and cover.
3. After that, let it sit until it reaches room temperature (about an hour or so). Then strain, pour into a jug and refrigerate.
4. Then, keep the 'stewed' apples – you can eat them as is, use them in chia pudding or porridge.
5. Finally, serve chilled during summer with fresh fruit.

Note: However, tried and tested, this makes for a beautiful hot tea during winter. Make sure to let it brew for about 10 minutes and enjoy with an extra sprinkle of cinnamon and turmeric.

Pineapple Beet Juice

Serves 1 (V, GF)

Ingredients

    1 small beet

    ¾" knob of ginger

    ½ pineapple (fresh)

    ½ cucumber

Directions:

1. First, remove the skin and core from the pineapple.
2. After which you cut into large chunks.
3. After that, put the chopped pineapple, cucumber, beet and ginger through a juicer.
4. Then, stir and enjoy.

Notes:

Organic produce is highly recommended for this recipe, if possible; otherwise, make sure to peel produce before juicing.

Blueberry yogurt protein smoothie

Serves 1

Ingredients

- 1 frozen banana (cut into chunks)
- ½ cup of quinoa flakes (or rolled oats)
- 1 cup of water
- 250g coconut yogurt
- 1 cup of blueberries
- small slice of lemon
- 2 Tablespoons of protein powder

To assemble: 2 Tablespoons of yogurt

Toppings: 1 teaspoon of puffed quinoa, fresh berries

Directions:

1. First, add all ingredients for the smoothie to a blender and blitz until smooth.
2. After which you add 2 Tablespoons of yogurt in the bottom of a jar and spread on the sides.
3. After that, pour smoothie in the jar.
4. Finally, add toppings and enjoy!

Mint, ginger and citrus green smoothie

Prep time: 2 minutes

Serves: 1

Ingredients

- 1 frozen banana (chopped)
- 1 mandarin or orange (pitted)
- 1 slice of ginger
- 3 small kale leaves
- 1/3 cups of coconut flakes/shreds
- 1 teaspoon of spirulina
- 1 cup of water
- 1 apple (chopped)
- 3 lemon slices
- Small handful of mint
- ½ cup of rolled oats
- 1 Tablespoon of chia seeds

For the middle layer: ½ cup puffed quinoa or buckwheat + 1/3 cup of coconut shreds/flakes

Toppings of choice (**NOTE:** I prefer coconut and frozen blueberries)

Directions:

1. First, add everything to a blender and process until it becomes very smooth.
2. After which you pour half in a jar, add the puffed quinoa and coconut flakes/shreds, then pour the remaining half.
3. Finally, add toppings and enjoy fresh!

Kale and passion fruit smoothie

Prep time: 5 mins

Serves: 1-2

Ingredients

- 1 small apple (cored)
- 1 passion fruit
- 1 frozen banana
- 1 ½ to 2 cups water
- 2-3 kale leaves
- 1 orange (peeled and pitted)
- Handful of cashews
- 1 lemon cube (**NOTE:** I freeze lemon juice in ice cube trays – alternatively you can use an ice cube and lemon juice)
- Optional: 1 teaspoon of bee pollen
- Top with (super)foods of choice

Directions:

First, chuck all ingredients to a blender and blitz until you get them smooth.

Anti-inflammatory fruit boost infused with rosemary

Prep time: 5 mins

Serves: 1-2

Ingredients

- 1 apple (roughly sliced)
- 1 small frozen banana
- 1 cm piece of ginger
- 1 Tablespoon of ground linseed
- 2 cups of water
- 1 orange (peeled and pitted)
- A good handful of strawberries
- 1 lemon cube (NOTE: I freeze lemon juice in ice cube trays)
- 1 teaspoon of turmeric powder
- 1 Tablespoon of chia seeds
- **Optional:** 1 teaspoon of bee pollen
- To serve: rosemary and toppings of choice

Directions:

1. First, chuck all to blender and whiz it good.
2. Then, use rosemary to stir things up.

Simple match a latte {dairy & sugar free}

Prep time: 5 mins

Serves: 1

Ingredients

- 1 cup of nut milk of choice (almond, macadamia, cashew milk)
- 1 teaspoon of match a green tea powder
- 1 (or 2) Tablespoons sweetener of choice (maple syrup, honey, agave)
- It is optional for a bit of extra energy and B vitamins: 1 teaspoon of bee pollen

Directions:

First, add all to blender and whiz until it becomes frothy and slightly warm.

Notes

1. However, if you don't have any nut milk lying around, I suggest you add 1/3 cup nuts of choice and 1 cup water to your blender and whiz for few seconds until you get milk.
2. On the other hand, strain it to remove some of the grainy pulp and then return the milk to the blender and make your match a latte.

Kale loquat green smoothie

Cook time: 5 mins

Serves: 1-2

Ingredients

> 1 banana
>
> Handful of loquats, pitted (**NOTE:** as far as I know, pits are slightly poisonous)
>
> 1 – 1 ½ cups water (or more, as needed to make a smooth concoction)
>
> 1 big kale leaf
>
> 1 apple (cored)
>
> 4-5 Tablespoons of lemon juice
>
> It is optional: ice cubes
>
> It is optional: bee pollen, chia seeds

Directions:

First, add all to blender and whiz up.

www.ingramcontent.com/pod-product-compliance
Lightning Source LLC
Chambersburg PA
CBHW081750100526
44592CB00015B/2366